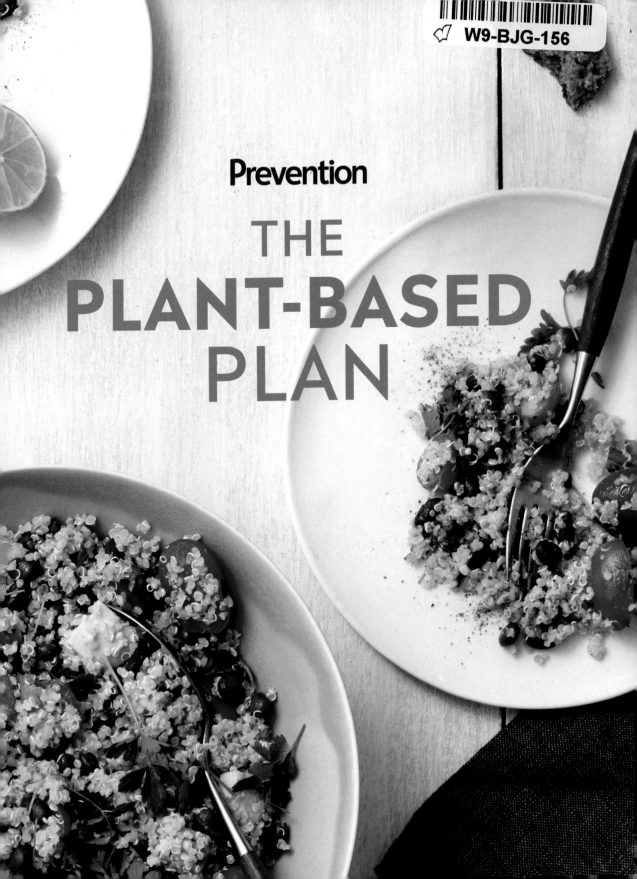

Prevention

THE
PLANT-BASED
PLAN

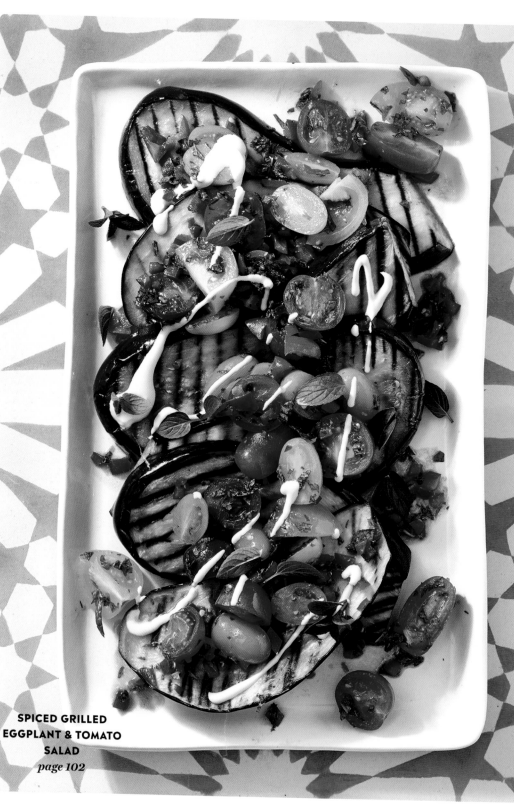

**SPICED GRILLED
EGGPLANT & TOMATO
SALAD**
page 102

Prevention

THE
PLANT-BASED
PLAN

TRANSFORM THE WAY YOU EAT

Preface by Joan Salge Blake, RDN

Foreword by Wendy Bazilian, DrPH, RDN

HEARST
HOME

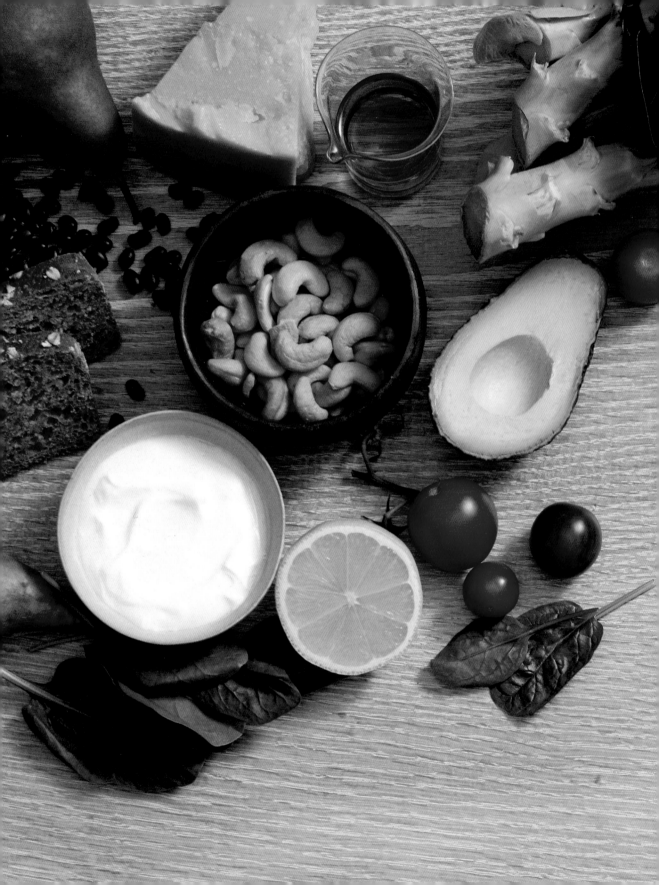

CONTENTS

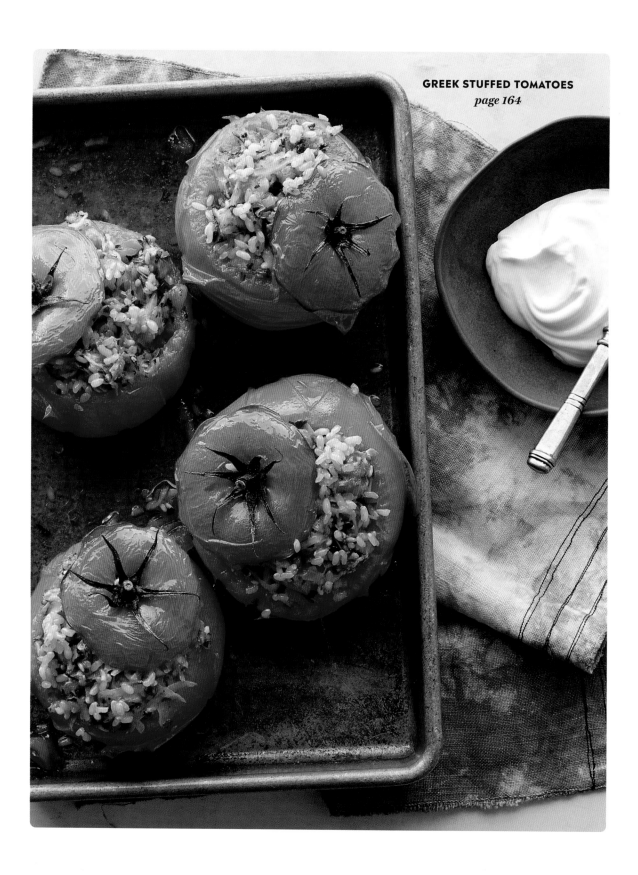

GREEK STUFFED TOMATOES
page 164

PREFACE

Never before has the adage "you are what you eat" held truer than right now. About half of American adults (117 million) have one or more preventable chronic diseases. Luckily, four of the top seven leading causes of death among Americans—namely, heart disease, certain cancers, stroke, and type 2 diabetes—can all be fought with a *knife and fork*. That is empowering.

Compelling research supports that a plant-forward diet—robust with vegetables, fruit, and whole grains, and prepared or even drizzled with healthy oils—along with adequate amounts of lean protein and dairy sources will improve your health and longevity. Bonus: You may find that you lose some weight too.

Many Americans are cooking at home more often and relying less on restaurant and takeout meals. This is good news: Research has shown that when we prepare more of our meals in the home, we reduce our consumption of heart-unhealthy saturated fat, sodium, and added sugars and increase consumption of heart- and waist-friendly fruits and vegetables. This is a *double* win.

People are hungry for healthy, delicious recipes that can be made in a snap. In a 2020 consumer survey conducted by the Food Industry Association, respondents agreed that eating at home is healthier but also shared what's most important to them when it comes to making that happen:

- convenience (meals that assemble quickly)
- health (nutritious, minimally processed foods)
- personal pleasure (taste, creativity, social connection)

The *Plant-Based Plan* puts all of these priorities in your reach, with more than 100 healthy and flavorful, easy recipes. This is a *triple* win.

Remember, you *are* what you eat, and what you eat can lead to a healthier, longer life. Enjoy.

—Joan Salge Blake, EdD, RDN, FAND, nutrition professor at Boston University
and host of the nutrition, health, and wellness podcast *Spot On!*

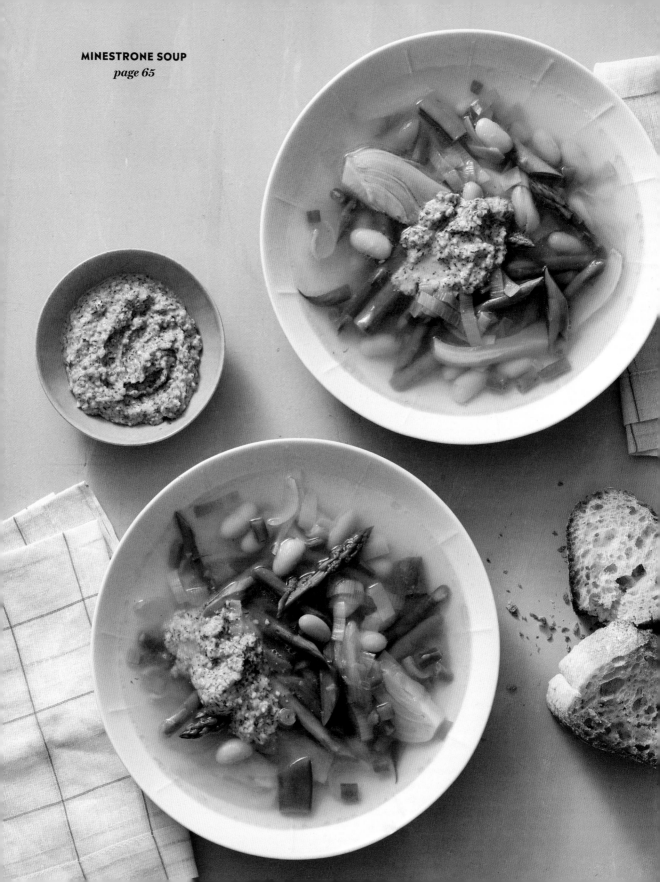

MINESTRONE SOUP
page 65

FOREWORD

We face a sea of choices when it comes to our food, and it can seem that the tide shifts rapidly. The latest, newest, and shiniest spin on what to eat is frequently complicated with restrictive rules and a long list of foods to avoid. It can be tricky to navigate and frustrating at times to find a way to eat healthier that fits *your* preferences, *your* style, and *your* personal goals.

Plant-based eating offers flexibility and simplicity along with science-backed benefits and fits right into your multitasking life, whether you are an active parent or have limited time to make home-cooked meals. Plus, once you know how to start, you'll find plant-based eating to be both delicious and sustainable. Plant-based eating is *the* recipe for better health.

Plus, it has actually been around for centuries (see page 13 for a brief history!). While it's not new, plant-based eating has suddenly become popular. But don't confuse it with one of those new, shiny fad diets. The fact is, it's the real deal.

In this book, *Prevention*'s trusted health editors offer approachable ways to incorporate plant-based eating into your life, whether you are starting out, already enjoy plant-based meals and would like to go a little further, or want to make a major commitment to plant-based eating at every meal. Plus, *Prevention*'s test kitchen chefs have created easy, flavorful (and nutritious!) plant-based recipes that you will actually make. And make again!

Ultimately, it's all about *more*. Plant-based eating simply means putting more plant foods on your plate—whether from vegetables, grains, legumes, nuts, or fruit. This book will be your road map to make that happen.

As a doctor of public health and registered dietitian, I know the science behind the benefits of plant-based eating and I've also seen this approach work well with many of my clients. One mom of three credited the "return" of her energy to plant-based eating. Another client found that her menopausal symptoms disappeared after only a few short weeks of consciously shifting toward a plant-based eating style. The benefits may vary, but they will add up—and show up—in your own life too. Enjoy your journey to more: more plants, more satisfaction, and more years of good health.

—Wendy Bazilian, DrPH, MA, RDN, educator and award-winning journalist

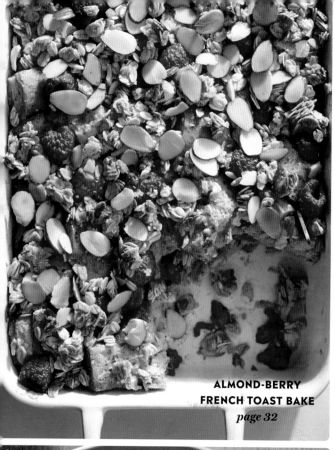

**ALMOND-BERRY
FRENCH TOAST BAKE**
page 32

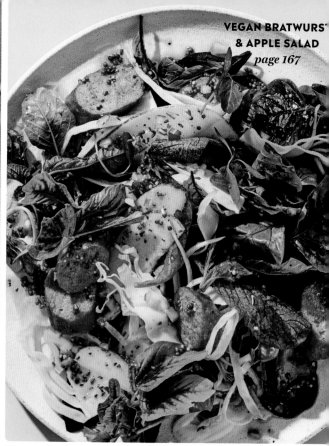

VEGAN BRATWURS*
& APPLE SALAD
page 167

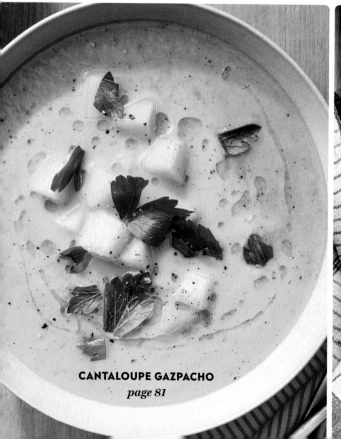

CANTALOUPE GAZPACHO
page 81

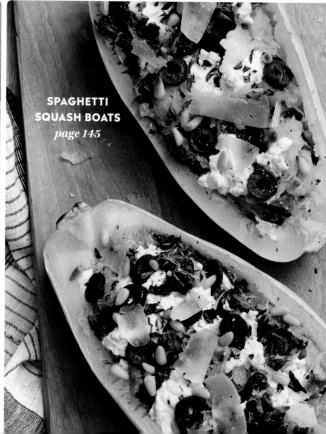

**SPAGHETTI
SQUASH BOATS**
page 145

INTRODUCTION

What Is a Plant-Based Diet?

More than ever before, there seems to be so many dietary buzzwords vegan, pescatarian, flexitarian, keto, paleo, fruitarian, lacto-ovo vegetarian—the list goes on. If there's one worth understanding and even adopting into your own diet, it's plant-based eating. Here's why.

Simply put, plant-based eating offers a set of guidelines that encourages eating more vegetables, fruits, and grains and less meat. "There's really not any one definition of what plant-based is," says Diana Sugiuchi, RDN, LDN, founder of Nourish Family Nutrition. "For some people, that means no meat; for some, that means a little bit of meat; and for some, that means adding in more plants." However, what all plant-based approaches have in common is the focus on eating *more* plants.

Plant-based eating differs from the Standard American Diet, which has long featured a sizable portion of meat as the star ingredient on a plate along with a large amount of a starchy dish, such as mac 'n' cheese or buttery mashed potatoes, and only a few vegetables scattered on the side. Our overall meat consumption proves it: Americans eat more meat than almost anyone else on the planet—around 53 pounds of pork, 58 pounds of beef, and 110 pounds of poultry per person per year. (To compare, other meat eaters around the world consume an average of 14 pounds of pork, 24 pounds of beef, and 32 pounds of poultry per person per year.) Many of us can't imagine a meal that doesn't feature some kind of animal product, yet we know that plant-based diets confer health benefits that a meat-heavy meal regimen does not.

But it's not all or nothing. Plant-based eating switches things around to make plants, not meat, the main feature of every meal—and it doesn't require giving up meat entirely. Whole foods grown from the earth, such as vegetables, fruits, beans, nuts, and whole grains, move front and center, while food derived from animals, such as beef, poultry, fish, and dairy, play more of a supporting role. "The emphasis is mostly on the vegetables and fruits, but you may also include foods like chicken or seafood every once in a while," says Jerlyn Jones, RDN, LD, owner of The Lifestyle Dietitian, an Atlanta-based nutrition consulting practice.

Plant-based eating is entirely customizable. For example, vegan and vegetarian diets are entirely plant-based. If those are too extreme for you, you can follow a plant-based plan and still eat animal products such as meat and dairy in moderation. You don't even need to worry about adhering to any one way of eating. "People want to put labels on the way they're eating: vegan, vegetarian, pescatarian," Sugiuchi says. "I'm much more a fan of being flexible, especially if you're transitioning into a different way of eating." When you know exactly what you want on your plate—more plants—there's no reason to strictly define your eating habits.

Ultimately, the way you go about eating more plant-based foods is up to you. Whether you decide to never eat meat or other animal products or have them only occasionally, plant-based eating empowers you to decide how you and your family will harness the power of plants.

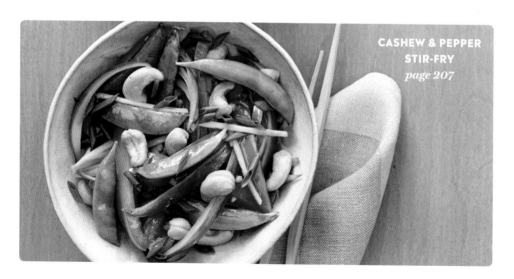

CASHEW & PEPPER
STIR-FRY
page 207

A PLANT-BASED HISTORY

Although plant-based seems like a relatively new way of eating, its principles are certainly not. "It's simply a new label for an eating style that has been around forever," says Wendy Bazilian, DrPH, RDN. For example, the Greek philosopher Pythagoras advocated for meatless diets in the 6th century BC, and vegetarian eating was called the "Pythagorean diet" until the mid-19th century. Plant-based eating was also popular among the thinkers of the Enlightenment, and Benjamin Franklin followed a plant-based diet. Plus, plenty of well-accepted and praised diets, including the centuries-old Mediterranean diet, are largely plant-based. Vegetarian eating finally reached the American mainstream in the 1970s, and it's only grown more popular since then. More recently, veganism, a diet that eliminates all animal products, has been growing significantly in popularity.

WHAT ARE THE HEALTH BENEFITS OF PLANT-BASED EATING?

Not all plant-based diets are equal. You can eat potato chips, white rice, and carrot cake every day and call it plant-based, but that won't benefit your overall health. In fact, one significant study from the American College of Cardiology found that while a plant-based diet focused on whole grains, fruits, and vegetables significantly lowered the risk of cardiovascular disease, a "plant-based" diet that included high-sugar, high-fat, processed foods (such as sweets and soda) plus refined grains and potatoes, had the opposite effect. If you're interested in plant-based eating because of its known health benefits, it's important to choose nutritionally balanced and healthful foods—that are also delicious!

Whole vegetables, fruits, and grains will have the most positive impact on your health because they're packed with vitamins, minerals, and nutrients. Plants are also the only source of phytonutrients, which are tens of thousands of unique compounds that work with other essential nutrients to improve overall health. Vegetables are high in nutrients and low in calories, "plus they can bring higher satiety due to nutrients and volume, so you don't have those energy highs and lows, and you don't get as many cravings," Bazilian explains.

"Everyone can benefit from eating more plant-based foods," Jones says. "It's not limited to only those who want to prevent or treat certain diseases." If you eat the plant-based foods you know are healthy, the benefits can include:

- A lower risk of developing type 2 diabetes

- A lower risk of heart disease

- A lower risk of developing cancer

- A lower rate of cognitive decline

- A better chance of weight loss

- A lower risk of obesity

ARE THERE OTHER BENEFITS TO A PLANT-BASED DIET?

Not only is plant-based eating good for your health, but it's good for the planet too. If you're concerned with the alarming news about climate change, switching to a plant-based diet can help shrink your carbon footprint. A landmark 2018 study reports that producing animal products takes up 83 percent of the world's farmland while producing only 18 percent of its calories. In other words, it's incredibly inefficient. Beef, in particular, is the worst offender: Producing 100 grams of beef protein (or less than 4 ounces, the average burger size) can emit 28 kilograms of greenhouse gas.

"If every American, on average, cut the equivalent of a burger out of their diet per week, it would be the equivalent of taking 10 million cars off the road each year," says Sujatha Bergen, director of health campaigns at the National Resources Defense Council. According to the same study, "dietary change can deliver environmental benefits on a scale not achievable by producers." Plant-based eating can make a tangible difference by cutting down on emissions, slowing deforestation, and encouraging responsible land use.

Another 2019 study in the *Proceedings of the National Academy of Science* ties together the health and environmental benefits: "Foods associated with the largest negative environmental impacts—unprocessed and processed red meat—are consistently associated with the largest increases in disease risk. Thus, dietary transitions toward greater consumption of healthier foods would generally improve environmental sustainability."

WHAT SHOULD I EAT ON A PLANT-BASED DIET?

Plant-based eating can be adapted to each person's tastes and needs. That said, the most impactful change to make when considering a plant-based diet is to reprioritize the food groups on your plate. Plant-based meals should consist of at least 75 percent plant-derived foods, according to health authorities such as Harvard Medical School. Harvard's guidelines suggest that the ideal plate—even for breakfast—should be composed of one-half vegetables and fruits and a quarter whole grains, such as quinoa, spelt, or rice. The last quarter is reserved for proteins, which can come from plants or animal products. Lean meats and dairy products are OK in moderation and can be considered an addition or side rather than the main event. (A few shrimp on top of a salad? Great! An 8-ounce steak with a side of veggies? Nope.)

If you are concerned about meeting your daily protein needs on a plant-based diet, rest assured there are many protein-packed plant-based foods available (see the list on page 16). Plus, there are plenty of nutrient-dense plant-based carbohydrates that work as amazing sources of energy. In fact, several world-class athletes—including arguably one of the most powerful of them all, Serena Williams—thrive on vegan or plant-based diets.

GET TO KNOW THE FOOD GROUPS

On the most basic level, food is categorized into five main groups: vegetables, fruits, grains, proteins, and dairy. Plant-based eating emphasizes the first four categories. Some researchers suggest that there should be more than five food groups—sometimes up to nine, which are further subdivided by nutritional content—but these five core groups are a good starting point when composing a balanced meal.

HOW DO I START?

Finding plant-based foods that you like is a culinary exploration. It's a chance to get out of eating (and cooking!) ruts and wake up your taste buds to a whole new world of flavor. Instead of sticking with romaine lettuce, for example, try customizing your salads with arugula, butterhead, or Little Gem. Or add varieties of peppers, onions, and mushrooms into your tacos and stir-fries. Think beyond white rice and instead use whole-grain brown rice, other seeds and grains such as quinoa (it's actually a seed!), and nutty and protein-packed farro. You'll find recipes throughout this book to help you do just that.

Think about the foods you eat now and evaluate them for the nutrients they include or the benefits they provide. Food should taste good, yes, but it should also work for you, making you feel healthy and satisfied. If some of your go-tos seem a little lacking, then swap them out for some of the easy recipes in this book. Another key to a successful plant-based diet is diversity: A growing body of research suggests that diets that include a variety of food groups are associated with lower rates of depression, osteoporosis, type 2 diabetes, and even death overall.

Almost all of the recipes in this book are vegetarian, and many are even vegan. (Vegan recipes will be marked with a 🌱.) They offer inspiration and delicious new ways to include more plant-based foods in your meals.

PROTEIN-PACKED PLANT-BASED FOODS

- Black beans, 7 grams per ½ cup
- Chickpeas, 7 grams per ½ cup
- Edamame, 12 grams per ⅔ cup
- Peanut butter, 7 grams per 2 tablespoons
- Quinoa, 8 grams per ¼ cup

- Steel-cut oats, 4 grams per ½ cup
- Tempeh, 16 grams per 3 ounces
- Tofu, 13 grams per 3 ounces
- Walnuts, 4 grams per ¼ cup

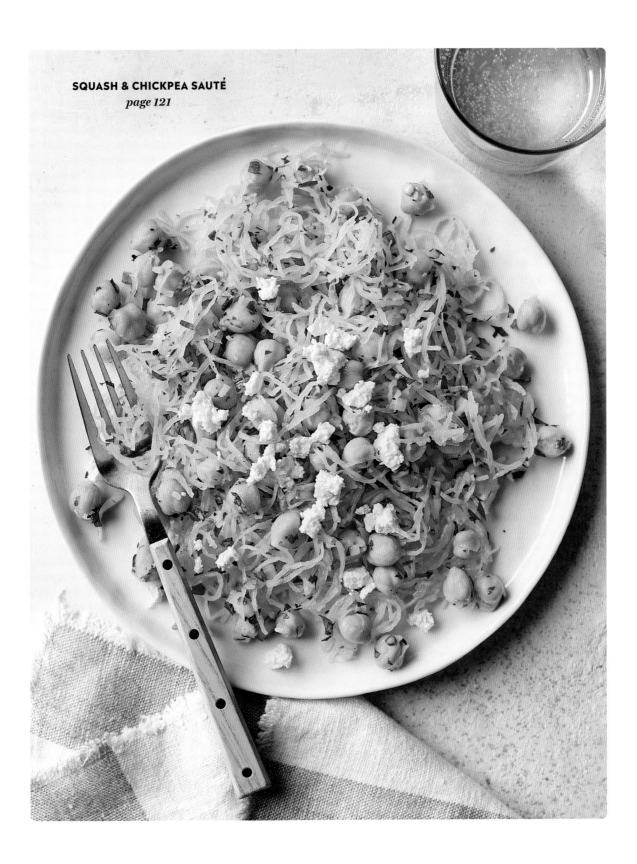

SQUASH & CHICKPEA SAUTÉ
page 121

The Prevention Plant-Based Plan

Our Plant-Based Plan offers a structured way to get started on your path to better health. It's based on three distinct levels of commitment, all customizable for your own needs. New to this? We suggest you start with level one. Looking for incorporate more plant-based meals into your daily meal rotation? Consider level two or three. But wherever you start, you will reap the benefits. "Transition to a plant-based diet step-by-step, and you'll find it's actually easy," Bazilian says. "It's a no-risk proposition." Let's get started!

1 Level One

ONE PLANT-BASED DAY OR THREE PLANT-BASED MEALS PER WEEK.

Level One presents to the basics of plant-based eating, and eases you into making a more substantial change if you choose.

"If you're eating a lot of meat," Sugiuchi says, "a meatless day, like the concept of Meatless Mondays, can be a great way to introduce these meals that feature less animal protein." Studies show that reducing the amount of animal products you eat can work wonders, from lowering the risk of cardiovascular disease to charging up metabolism. You can reap these rewards from one plant-based day a week or by having three plant-based dishes throughout the week.

To reduce the amount of meat you eat, aim for no more than 24 ounces of cooked meat per week (just over 3 ounces, or about one palm-size serving, per day), a serving size recommended by the American Heart Association and the American Cancer Society, among other authorities. When you have less meat on your plate, you will have more room for filling and satisfying plant-based foods.

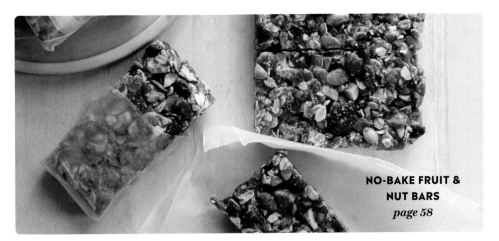

**NO-BAKE FRUIT &
NUT BARS**
page 58

2 Level Two

THREE PLANT-BASED DAYS OR NINE PLANT-BASED MEALS PER WEEK.

Once you're a bit more familiar with plant-based food, Level Two is where you might start to get out of your comfort zone (in a good way, of course). Three days should be devoted entirely to plant-based eating or instead, you can prepare nine plant-based recipes to have throughout the week—it's your choice.

You may start to notice some growing pains here, but that's part of the process: "It's not always easy for people to initially cut back on the amount of animal products they consume," says Brian Kateman, president and cofounder of the Reducetarian Foundation, an organization that advocates for reducing animal products in your diet. "They have to be patient with themselves and patient with those who are trying around them. Beginning that process—viewing each meal as an opportunity to make a better choice—is definitely something that is doable."

Another goal in this stage of plant-based eating is reducing your animal products to 18 ounces a week. With a variety of replacements for animal proteins on the market such as plant-based burgers, sausages, and more, you may not even miss them.

3 Level Three

FIVE PLANT-BASED DAYS OR 15 PLANT-BASED MEALS PER WEEK.

This level is for plant-loving devotees who are ready to increase their commitment. If you're feeling particularly ambitious, you can even decide to switch to 100-percent plant-powered eating—this book has more than enough recipes for you to do so.

This stage is when you might start to notice more of the perks of eating mostly plants, including the ones listed on page 14. One recent review of more than 30 studies on plant-based eating found many short- and long-term benefits for overall health, including increased metabolism, decreased inflammation, and easier weight loss.

At Level Three, we suggest eating no more than 9 ounces of meat and poultry each week. That's still plenty to enjoy on those special occasions— such as barbecues, game-night nachos, and Thanksgiving turkey—or and an evening when you simply crave a burger without feeling restricted.

THE SIMPLEST WAY TO START

This journey might be challenging, but it's almost guaranteed to be rewarding. Instead of establishing one entirely plant-based day, try adding more plants to meals you already love, Bazilian suggests. "There are 21 meals in a week, so begin by adding fruits or vegetables to one a day. For example, if you eat eggs and toast for breakfast, add salsa, spinach, or avocado. If you add a soup or salad to your lunch or dinner every day, you'll be getting nutrient-dense vegetables."

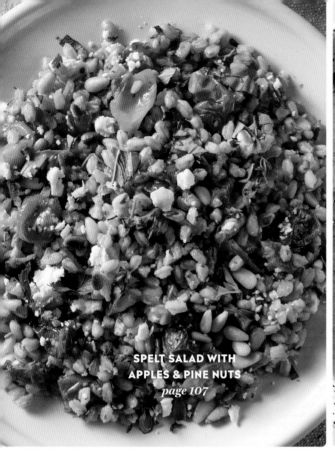

**SPELT SALAD WITH
APPLES & PINE NUTS**
page 107

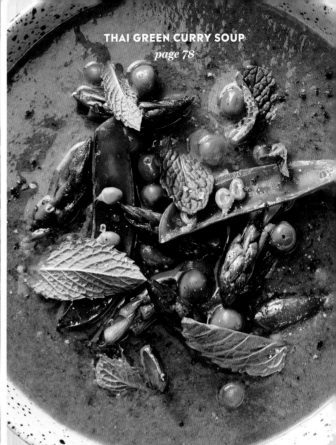

THAI GREEN CURRY SOUP
page 78

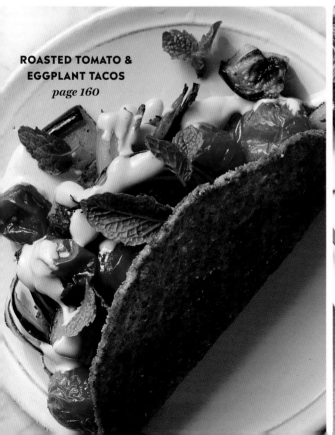

**ROASTED TOMATO &
EGGPLANT TACOS**
page 160

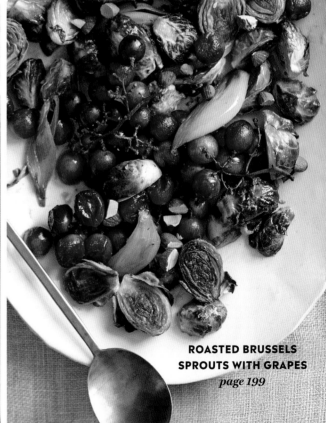

**ROASTED BRUSSELS
SPROUTS WITH GRAPES**
page 199

A WEEK OF PLANT-BASED EATING

Need some inspiration for your days of plant-based eating? Check out this seven-day menu to help get you started. Mix and match the meals and menus that most appeal to you.

Day 1

BREAKFAST Butternut Squash & Spinach Toasts (page 54)

LUNCH Blueberry-Arugula Salad with Dijon Vinaigrette (page 98)

DINNER Tofu, Lentil & Swiss Chard Tacos (page 153)

SNACK Mango Rolls (page 184)

Day 2

BREAKFAST Veggie-Loaded Chickpea Waffles (page 35)

LUNCH Southwestern Chopped Salad (page 91)

DINNER Butternut Squash & Mole Enchiladas (page 172)

SNACK Eggplant & Zucchini Fries with Roasted Tomato Dip (page 211)

Day 3

BREAKFAST Harissa & Egg Brunch Pizza (page 27)

LUNCH Minestrone Soup (page 65)

DINNER Guava Barbecue Sauce & Pulled Jackfruit Sandwich (page 148)

SNACK Corn on the Cob with Chili-Lime Sauce (page 204)

Day 4

BREAKFAST Cranberry-Banana Smoothie (page 41)

LUNCH Greek Chickpea Tacos (page 132)

DINNER Asian Tofu with Baby Bok Choy (page 156)

SNACK: Blistered Sugar Snap Peas (page 183)

Day 5

BREAKFAST Spring Radish & Avocado Toast (page 57)

LUNCH Kale Caesar Salad (page 101)

DINNER Rigatoni with Pistachio Pesto (page 114)

SNACK Maple-Roasted Beets (page 188)

Day 6

BREAKFAST No-Syrup Pancakes (page 36)

LUNCH Lentil-Broccoli Falafel Bowl with Jalapeño-Herb Tahini (page 176)

DINNER Farro Risotto with Fennel, Peas & Greens (page 141)

SNACK "Cheesy" Kale Chips (page 197)

Day 7

BREAKFAST Almond-Berry French Toast Bake (page 32)

LUNCH Corn, Mango & Edamame Salad (page 94)

DINNER Greek Stuffed Tomatoes (page 164)

SNACK: Roasted Veggies with Olive Dressing (page 200)

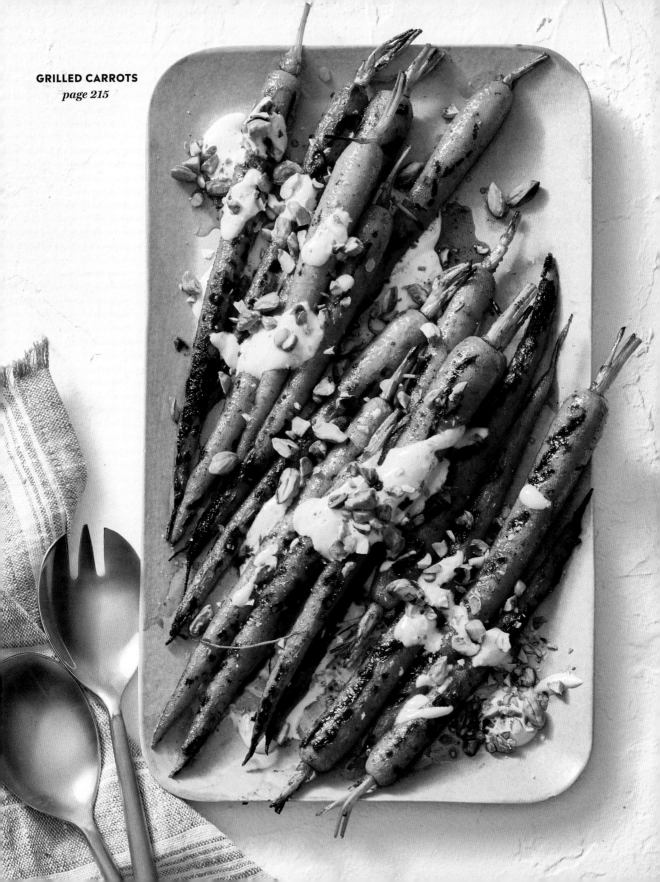

GRILLED CARROTS
page 215

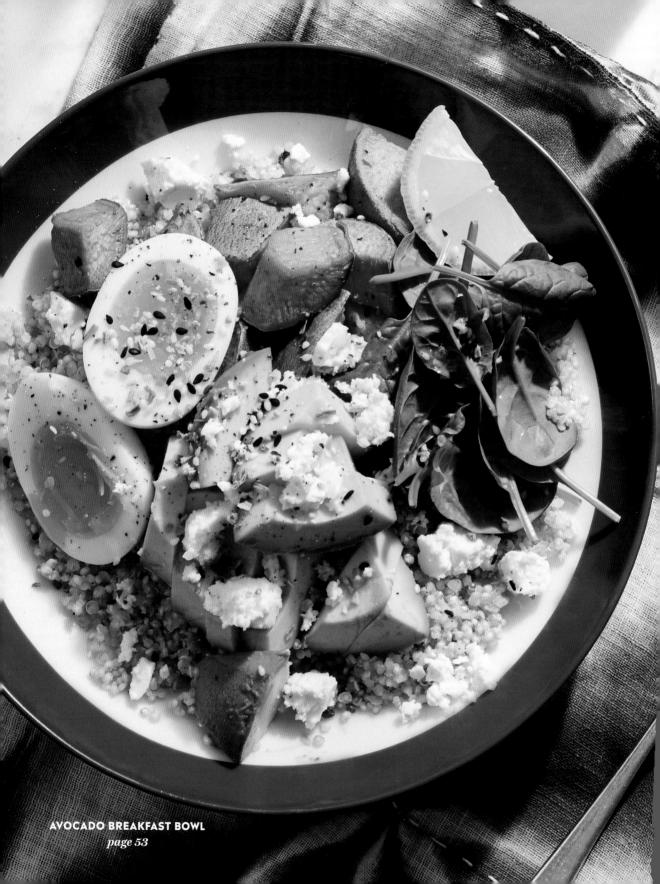

AVOCADO BREAKFAST BOWL
page 53

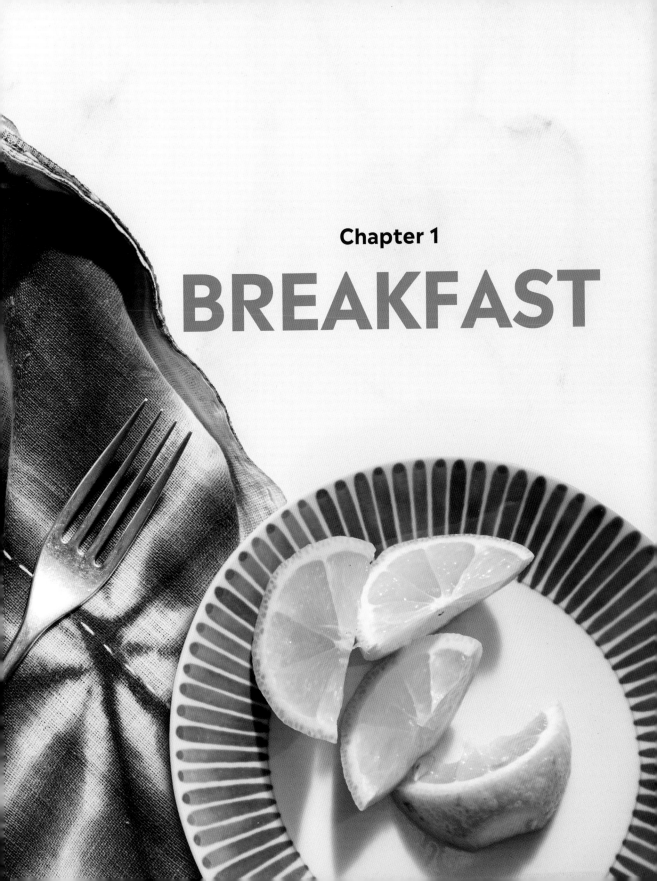

Chapter 1
BREAKFAST

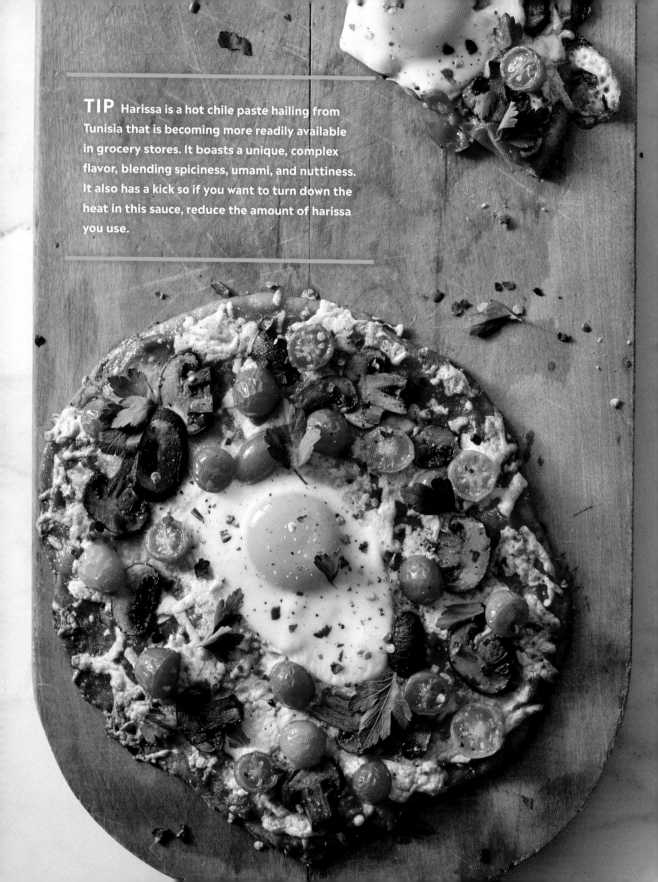

TIP Harissa is a hot chile paste hailing from Tunisia that is becoming more readily available in grocery stores. It boasts a unique, complex flavor, blending spiciness, umami, and nuttiness. It also has a kick so if you want to turn down the heat in this sauce, reduce the amount of harissa you use.

HARISSA & EGG BRUNCH PIZZA

TOTAL TIME: 35 MINUTES ◆ SERVES 6

This shakshuka-inspired personal pizza brightens up the meat-and-cheese-heavy classic with a hefty dose of mushrooms, fresh tomatoes, and, of course, sunny-side up eggs. The tomatoes are rich in lycopene, which has been linked to lowering cancer and heart disease risk.

Cooking spray

½ cup marinara sauce

½ cup harissa

2 teaspoons ground cumin

All-purpose flour

1 pound whole-wheat pizza dough, divided into 6 balls

6 ounces part-skim mozzarella, shredded

8 ounces heirloom cherry or grape tomatoes, halved (quartered if large)

3 ounces mushrooms, sliced

6 large eggs

¼ cup parsley, for topping

Red pepper flakes, for topping (optional)

1. Heat oven to 500°F. Coat 3 baking sheets with cooking spray and set aside. In a bowl, combine marinara, harissa, and cumin.

2. On lightly floured surface, roll dough into 6 rounds about 10 inches in diameter and ⅛-inch thick and place on the baking sheets. If dough shrinks, leave at room temperature 10 minutes and roll again.

3. Bake until dough is slightly puffed and set, about 5 minutes. Remove from oven. Spread marinara mixture over dough. Top with cheese, then tomatoes and mushrooms. Crack 1 egg over each pizza.

4. Return pan to oven and bake until egg is set and crust is golden, about 8 minutes. Serve topped with parsley and red pepper flakes, if desired.

PER SERVING 370 calories, 16.5 g fat (4.5 g saturated fat), 21 g protein, 815 mg sodium, 38 g carbohydrates, 6 g fiber, 1 g sugars (0 g added sugars), 204 mg cholesterol

SPINACH-CURRY CREPES WITH APPLE, RAISINS & CHICKPEAS

TOTAL TIME: 40 MINUTES ◆ SERVES 6

The French breakfast favorite gets a plant-based remix in this recipe, which combines fiber-rich apples, protein-packed chickpeas, and vitamin-C-loaded lemon into a savory-sweet treat.

2 large eggs

⅓ cup finely chopped cilantro

¼ teaspoon black pepper

2½ cups 1-percent milk, divided

1 cup plus 2 tablespoons all-purpose flour

3 tablespoons safflower oil, divided

¾ teaspoon kosher salt, divided

Cooking spray

1 small yellow onion, chopped

1 (15.5-ounce) can chickpeas, drained and rinsed

1 Granny Smith apple, diced

¼ cup golden raisins

2 tablespoons Madras curry powder

10 ounces spinach

Lemon wedges, for serving

1. In a blender, puree eggs, cilantro, pepper, 1 cup milk, 1 cup flour, 2 tablespoons oil, and ¼ teaspoon salt. Lightly coat a 10-inch nonstick skillet with cooking spray and place on medium heat.

2. Pour ⅓ cup batter into the pan, spreading it evenly across the surface. Cook until edges set, about 1 minute. Flip and cook 30 seconds. Remove from the pan and cover to keep warm. Repeat with remaining batter.

3. Heat remaining 1 tablespoon oil in a separate skillet on medium. Add onion and cook until soft, about 5 minutes. Add chickpeas, apples, raisins, and curry powder. Cook 3 minutes. Stir in remaining 2 tablespoons flour and cook 30 seconds. Stir in remaining 1½ cups milk. Cook until thick, about 2 minutes. Add spinach and remaining ½ teaspoon salt. Cook until wilted, about 2 minutes.

4. Divide chickpea mixture among crepes, fold each crepe in half, and serve with lemon wedges.

PER SERVING 325 calories, 11 g fat (2 g saturated fat), 13 g protein, 540 mg sodium, 47 g carbohydrates, 6 g fiber, 13 g sugars (0 g added sugars), 67 mg cholesterol

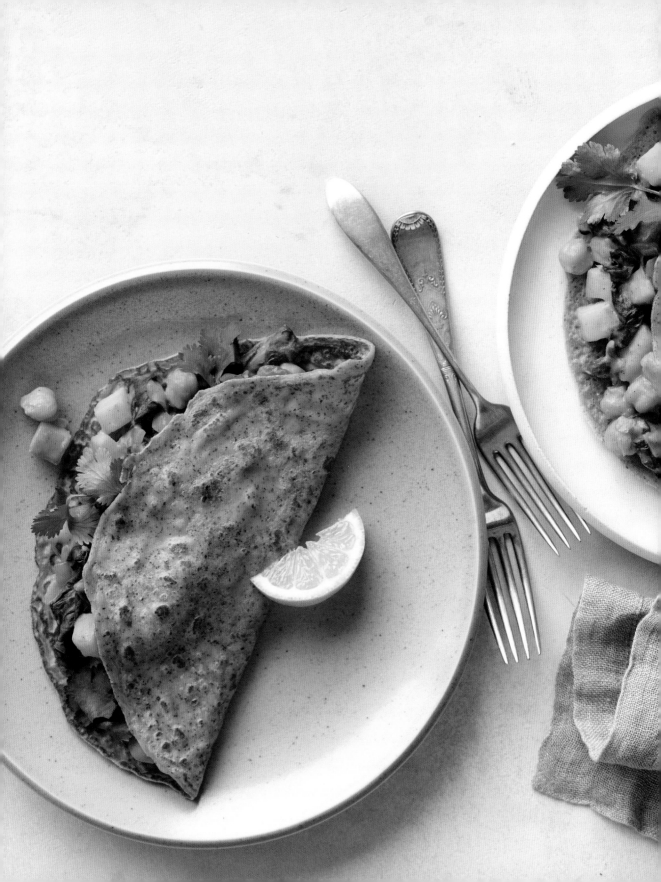

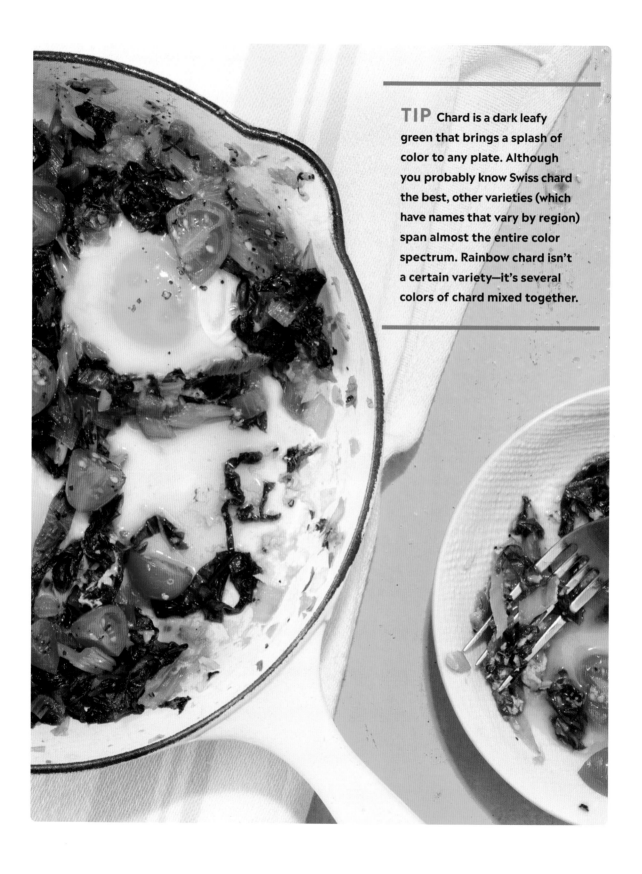

TIP Chard is a dark leafy green that brings a splash of color to any plate. Although you probably know Swiss chard the best, other varieties (which have names that vary by region) span almost the entire color spectrum. Rainbow chard isn't a certain variety—it's several colors of chard mixed together.

CHARD BREAKFAST SKILLET WITH EGG, ONION & TOMATO

TOTAL TIME: 30 MINUTES ◆ SERVES 4

Enjoy a guilt-free brunch with this skillet, which makes the most of nutrient-dense leafy greens without the bitter flavor. Chard is an especially great source of plant-based calcium, potassium, and vitamin C.

1¼ cups quartered cherry tomatoes

1 tablespoon red wine vinegar

2 bunches Swiss chard or rainbow chard

2 cups chopped yellow onion

3 tablespoons extra virgin olive oil

4 cloves garlic, minced

½ teaspoon sea salt

½ teaspoon ground black pepper

4 large eggs

1. In a small bowl, toss cherry tomatoes with vinegar. Set aside.

2. Remove chard leaves from stems. Chop leaves, place in a large bowl of cool water, and swirl to rinse. Transfer to a colander, allowing a bit of water to remain on leaves. Rinse, dry, and thinly slice stems.

3. In a large cast-iron skillet on medium heat, sauté chard stems and onion in oil until softened, about 10 minutes. Reduce heat to low. Add garlic and sauté 1 minute. Add chard leaves, salt, and pepper. Turn heat to high and toss with tongs until leaves wilt.

4. Using the back of a spoon, make 4 indentations, or "nests," in chard. Crack 1 egg into each nest. Cover the skillet, reduce heat slightly, and cook until yolks are medium-set, about 4 minutes.

5. Add cherry tomatoes and vinegar to skillet, then serve.

PER SERVING 245 calories, 16 g fat (3 g saturated fat), 11 g protein, 635 mg sodium, 17 g carbohydrates, 5 g fiber, 7 g sugars (0 g added sugars), 187 mg cholesterol

ALMOND-BERRY FRENCH TOAST BAKE

TOTAL TIME: 1 HOUR PLUS 3 HOURS CHILLING ◆ SERVES 9

Whole grains like those in whole-wheat bread provide higher amounts of protein and fiber, both of which slow the absorption of sugar in your bloodstream.

Cooking spray

12 slices stale whole-wheat bread, cut into 1½-inch cubes

6 to 8 ounces raspberries

6 large eggs

2 large egg whites

2¼ cups 2-percent milk

3 tablespoons maple syrup

2 teaspoons vanilla extract

¾ teaspoon cinnamon

½ teaspoon kosher salt

¼ cup rolled oats

¼ cup sliced almonds

1. Coat a 9-inch rectangular baking dish with cooking spray. Scatter bread cubes and berries in an even layer.

2. In a bowl, whisk together eggs, egg whites, milk, maple syrup, vanilla, cinnamon, and salt. Pour wet ingredients over bread cubes. Cover and chill for 3 hours. Sprinkle oats and almonds over top.

3. Heat oven to 350°F. Bake until puffed and golden, about 50 minutes.

PER SERVING 240 calories, 7.5 g fat (2 g saturated fat), 12 g protein, 345 mg sodium, 32 g carbohydrates, 6 g fiber, 13 g sugars (4 g added sugars), 130 mg cholesterol

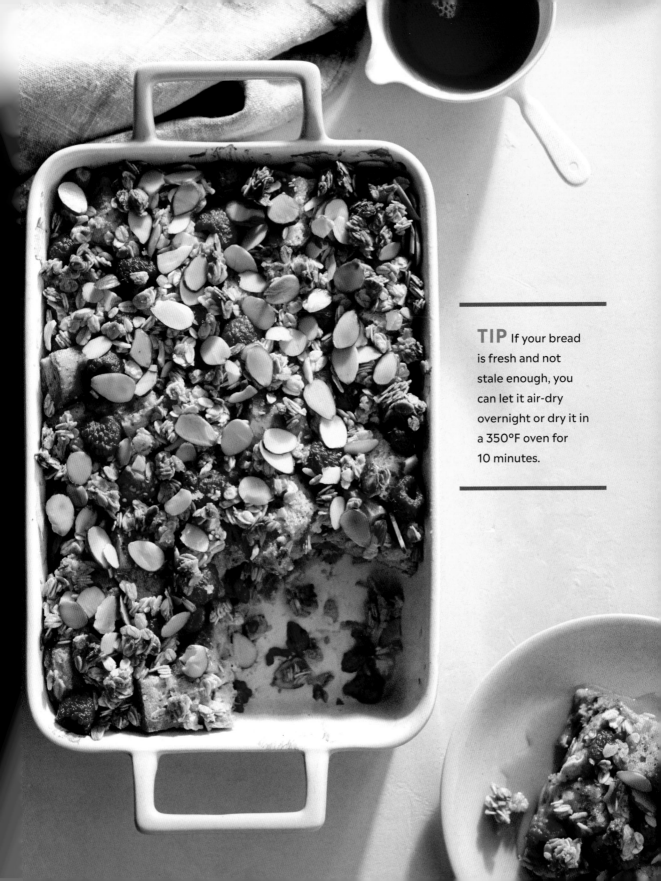

TIP If your bread is fresh and not stale enough, you can let it air-dry overnight or dry it in a 350°F oven for 10 minutes.

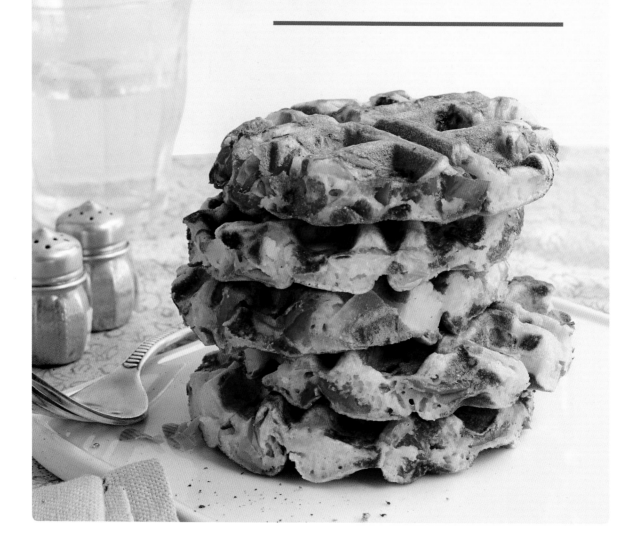

TIP When it comes to alternative flours, chickpea flour might be the one to beat them all. Nutty and not overpoweringly beany, it has a subtle sweetness that works well in both savory dishes and desserts. Plus, like whole chickpeas, chickpea flour is loaded with protein and fiber—20 grams of the former and 10 grams of the latter in each cup—to keep you satiated.

VEGGIE-LOADED CHICKPEA WAFFLES

TOTAL TIME: 15 MINUTES ◆ SERVES 8

Just one of these low-carb waffles packs more protein than an egg (at just 85 calories a pop, no less). Savor every veggie-loaded bite, avoid hitting a carb slump before noon, and feel full all morning long.

½ cup chickpea flour

¼ teaspoon baking soda

¼ teaspoon kosher salt

½ cup plain 2-percent Greek yogurt

4 large eggs

2 scallions, finely chopped

1 cup baby spinach, roughly chopped

½ small red pepper, cut into thin pieces

3 tablespoons grated Pecorino Romano cheese

¼ teaspoon black pepper

Cooking spray

1. Heat oven to 200°F. Set a wire rack over a rimmed baking sheet and place in oven. Heat waffle iron per appliance's directions.

2. In a large bowl, whisk together chickpea flour, baking soda, and salt. In a small bowl, whisk together yogurt and eggs. Stir wet ingredients into dry ingredients. Fold in scallions, spinach, red pepper, cheese, and black pepper.

3. Lightly coat waffle iron with cooking spray and, in batches, drop ¼ cup batter into each section of iron and cook until golden brown, 4 to 5 minutes. Transfer to the baking sheet in oven and keep warm. Repeat with remaining batter.

PER SERVING 85 calories, 4 g fat (1.5 g saturated fat), 7 g protein, 195 mg sodium, 5 g carbohydrates, 1 g fiber, 2 g sugars (0 g added sugars), 98 mg cholesterol

NO-SYRUP PANCAKES

TOTAL TIME: 25 MINUTES ◆ SERVES 4

Skip the syrup! These easy-to-make delights can be enjoyed alone. The apple slices cooked into these pancakes offer a rich, natural sweetness plus pectin, a soluble fiber that may help lower cholesterol.

1 cup all-purpose flour

2 teaspoons baking powder

½ teaspoon cinnamon

½ teaspoon salt

½ cup 2-percent milk

½ cup unsweetened applesauce

2 tablespoons unsalted butter, melted

1 large egg

Cooking spray

1 apple, peeled and thinly sliced into rounds

1. In a medium bowl, whisk together flour, baking powder, cinnamon, and salt.

2. In a large bowl, whisk together milk, applesauce, butter, and egg. Add dry ingredients and stir just until combined. (Batter should be slightly lumpy.)

3. Lightly coat a large skillet with cooking spray and heat on medium. Spoon ¼-cup portions of batter into the skillet and lightly push an apple slice into each.

4. Cook until bubbles appear at sides of pancakes, 1 to 2 minutes. Flip and cook until browned, 1 to 2 minutes more. Transfer to a plate and cover to keep warm. Repeat with remaining batter and apple slices.

PER SERVING 245 calories, 9 g fat (5 g saturated fat), 7 g protein, 635 mg sodium, 36 g carbohydrates, 2 g fiber, 10 g sugars (0 g added sugars), 67 mg cholesterol

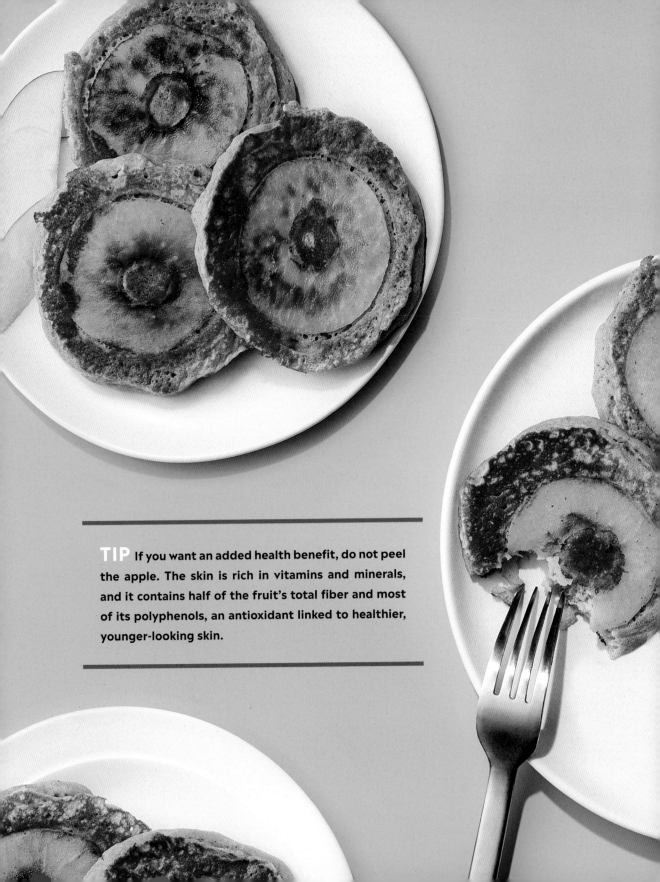

TIP If you want an added health benefit, do not peel the apple. The skin is rich in vitamins and minerals, and it contains half of the fruit's total fiber and most of its polyphenols, an antioxidant linked to healthier, younger-looking skin.

BROWN RICE PORRIDGE 🌱

TOTAL TIME: 15 MINUTES ◆ SERVES 1

This two-step porridge is almost too good to be true: It's packed with fiber, made with common pantry ingredients, and completely vegan. The pomegranate seeds, rich in vitamin C and potassium, also facilitate digestion.

½ cup cooked brown rice

⅓ cup coconut milk

⅛ teaspoon vanilla extract

¼ teaspoon cinnamon

¼ teaspoon salt

½ teaspoon maple syrup

¼ cup sliced pear

1 teaspoon pomegranate seeds

2 teaspoons coconut flakes

1. In a small saucepan, place cooked brown rice, ½ cup water, coconut milk, vanilla, cinnamon, and salt. Bring to a boil, lower heat, cover, and simmer 10 minutes.

2. Transfer to a bowl and top with maple syrup, pear, pomegranate seeds, and coconut flakes.

PER SERVING 315 calories, 19 g fat (16 g saturated fat), 10 g protein, 490 mg sodium, 34 g carbohydrates, 4 g fiber, 6 g sugars (2 g added sugars), 0 mg cholesterol

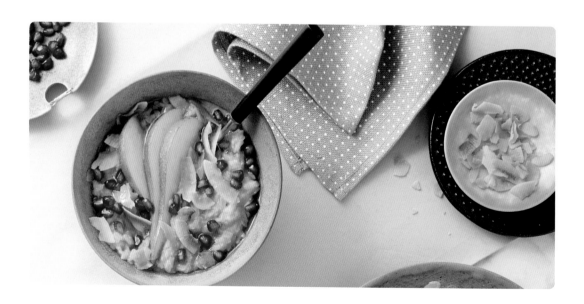

WHOLE-WHEAT CRANBERRY PROTEIN PANCAKE BITES

TOTAL TIME: 25 MINUTES ◆ SERVES 4

This grab-and-go morning meal is packed with the antioxidant-rich goodness of cranberries, which have been shown to improve digestion, prevent gum disease, and even boost your immune system.

1½ cups whole-wheat flour

½ cup quick-cooking oats

2 tablespoons protein powder

2 teaspoons baking powder

½ teaspoon cinnamon

¼ teaspoon kosher salt

1 large egg

1 cup unsweetened almond milk

¼ cup plain nonfat Greek yogurt

2 tablespoons pure maple syrup

1 teaspoon vanilla extract

½ cup cranberries, chopped (thawed if frozen)

1. In a large bowl, whisk together flour, oats, protein powder, baking powder, cinnamon, and salt.

2. In a medium bowl, whisk together egg, almond milk, yogurt, maple syrup, and vanilla. Gradually add wet ingredients to dry ones and whisk until smooth. Fold in cranberries.

3. Cook pancakes (about 2 tablespoons batter each) in a nonstick pan on medium until golden brown, about 3 minutes per side.

PER SERVING 285 calories, 4 g fat (1 g saturated fat), 14 g protein, 505 mg sodium, 50 g carbohydrates, 7 g fiber, 7.5 g sugars (6 g added sugars), 47 mg cholesterol

TIP Consider using a plant-based protein powder. Many popular protein powders are derived from dairy and include whey and casein. If you want to cut down on your animal product consumption, you can look for protein powders made from peas, soy, hemp, or other plants.

COCONUT-CHIA PUDDING 🌱

TOTAL TIME: 5 MINUTES PLUS 2 HOURS CHILLING ◆ SERVES 6

The secret to the texture in this creamy yet crunchy breakfast is tiny chia seeds, which are packed with major nutrients such as omega-3 fatty acids, calcium, magnesium, and more.

½ cup black chia seeds

3 tablespoons agave syrup

2 teaspoons vanilla extract

⅛ teaspoon kosher salt

1 (14-ounce) can light coconut milk, shaken

1 cup almond milk or other nondairy milk

Berries, for topping

Pepitas, for topping

1. In a large bowl, combine chia seeds, agave syrup, vanilla, and salt, making sure there are no clumps. Whisk in coconut and almond milks.

2. Transfer to a jar, cover, and refrigerate for at least 2 hours. Serve topped with berries and pepitas.

PER SERVING 255 calories, 19.5 g fat (12.5 g saturated fat), 4 g protein, 80 mg sodium, 17 g carbohydrates, 7 g fiber, 7 g sugars (7 g added sugars), 0 mg cholesterol

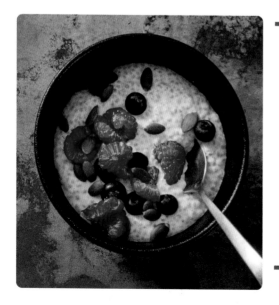

TIP Have leftover chia seeds? Turn them into raspberry-chia jam. In a small saucepan, cook **2 cups** raspberries on medium, stirring occasionally, until fruit breaks down and liquid becomes syrupy, about 8 minutes. Remove from heat and stir in **1 tablespoon each lemon juice and maple syrup**, then stir in **2 tablespoons chia seeds**. Let sit at least 20 minutes (the mixture should thicken slightly). Enjoy on whole-grain toast.

CRANBERRY-BANANA SMOOTHIE

TOTAL TIME: 5 MINUTES ◆ SERVES 1

Cranberries, the antioxidant-rich berry, make this smoothie both filling and low-calorie. To kick your breakfast up a notch, try adding a scoop of vegan protein powder to the mix, which will help you feel even more satisfied.

1 cup frozen cranberries

1 cup unsweetened almond milk

1 banana

1 tablespoon maple syrup

½ cup ice cubes

In a blender, puree cranberries, almond milk, banana, maple syrup, and ice cubes.

PER SERVING 125 calories, 1.5 g fat (0 g saturated fat), 1 g protein, 90 mg sodium, 27 g carbohydrates,4 g fiber, 15.5 g sugars (6 g added sugars), 0 mg cholesterol

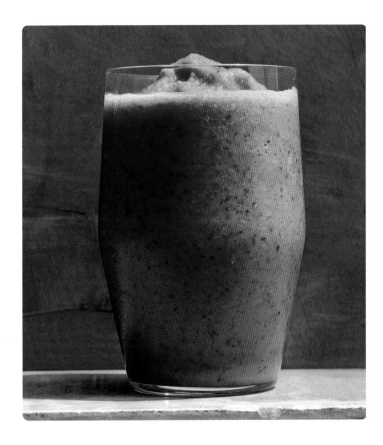

BLUEBERRY COBBLER SMOOTHIE BOWL 🌱

TOTAL TIME: 10 MINUTES ◆ SERVES 2

This bowl starts your day off right with 25 grams of protein to keep you full for hours, healthy fats to lower risk of a heart attack or stroke, and cinnamon to boost brainpower.

1 cup frozen blueberries

½ cup unsweetened almond milk

1½ scoops protein powder

2 tablespoons almond butter

1 teaspoon vanilla extract

½ cup blueberries

¼ cup vanilla granola

2 tablespoons sliced almonds

2 teaspoons hemp seeds

1 teaspoon cinnamon

1. In a blender, puree blueberries, almond milk, protein powder, almond butter, and vanilla extract until creamy. Divide between 2 bowls.

2. Top each bowl with blueberries, granola, almonds, hemp seeds, and cinnamon before serving.

PER SERVING 370 calories, 17 g fat (2.5 g saturated fat), 25 g protein, 130 mg sodium, 32 g carbohydrates, 7 g fiber, 16 g sugars (4 g added sugars), 0 mg cholesterol

SMART SMOOTHIE ADD-INS

Smoothie bowls can quickly become unhealthy if they're topped with ingredients that are high in sugar. These are five smart sprinkles we use.

Berries These gems are packed with disease-fighting antioxidants along with fiber to aid digestion and help you feel full faster.

Nuts They are rich sources of unsaturated fats, which reduce inflammation and lower the risk of heart disease, cancer, and arthritis.

Rolled Oats This whole grain contains beta-glucan, a type of fiber shown to cut cholesterol, control blood sugar, and help control inflammation.

Seeds The vitamin E in pumpkin and sunflower seeds strengthens the immune system to ramp up its defense against bacteria and viruses.

Dried Fruit Golden raisins contain more antioxidants than dark raisins. Goji berries are high in protein and immune-boosting vitamin C.

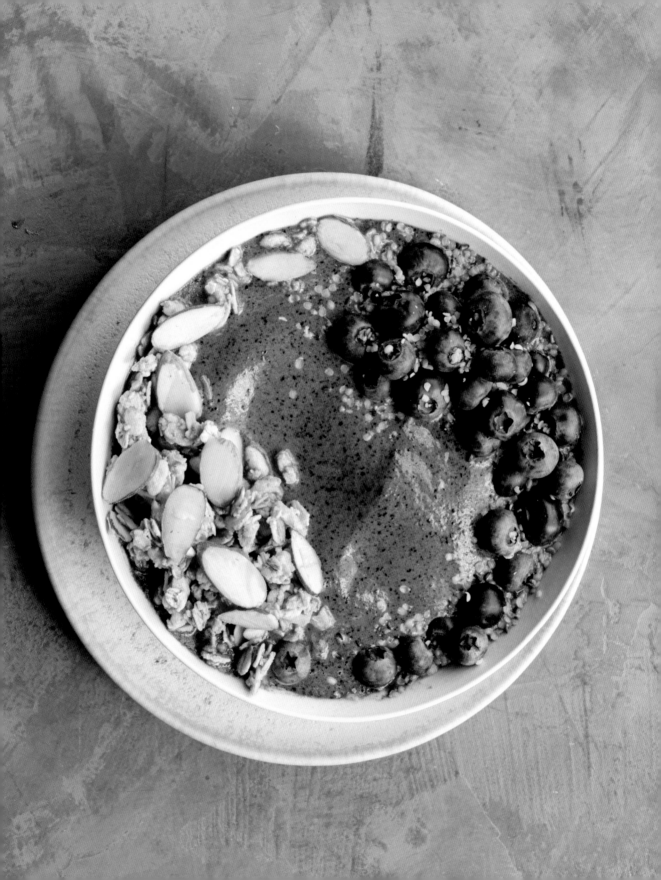

GOOD MORNING COFFEE SMOOTHIE ❧

TOTAL TIME: 5 MINUTES ◆ SERVES 1

Coffee and smoothies are morning staples, so why not combine the two into a delicious vegan blend? Plus, the caffeine in coffee stimulates muscles and thus aids in digestion.

1 cup unsweetened almond milk, coconut milk, or cashew milk

1 frozen banana

½ cup coffee, chilled

½ cup blueberries

2 tablespoons unsweetened cacao powder

¼ teaspoon cinnamon

In a blender, combine all ingredients. Blend until it reaches the desired consistency.

PER SERVING 215 calories, 6 g fat (1.5 g saturated fat), 5 g protein, 185 mg sodium, 45 g carbohydrates, 10 g fiber, 22 g sugars (0 g added sugars), 0 mg cholesterol

TIP For decades, patients with abnormal heart rhythms (which can increase the risk for sudden cardiac arrest and stroke) were advised to avoid caffeine. However, recent analysis indicates that drinking coffee can actually decrease atrial fibrillation frequency by up to 13 percent. Additionally, according to a *BMJ* review, people who drink coffee are 19 percent less likely to die of cardiovascular disease and 30 percent less likely to die of a stroke than their coffee-abstaining counterparts.

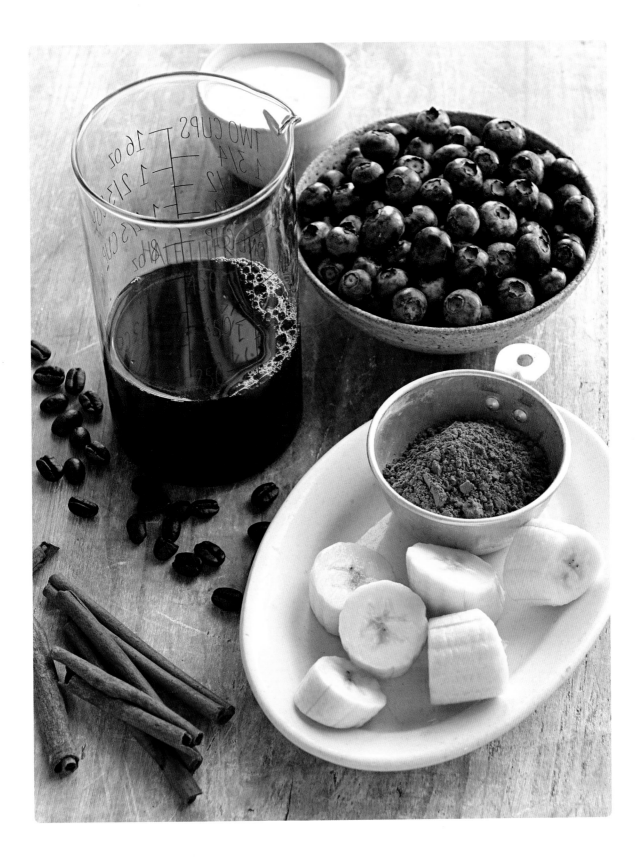

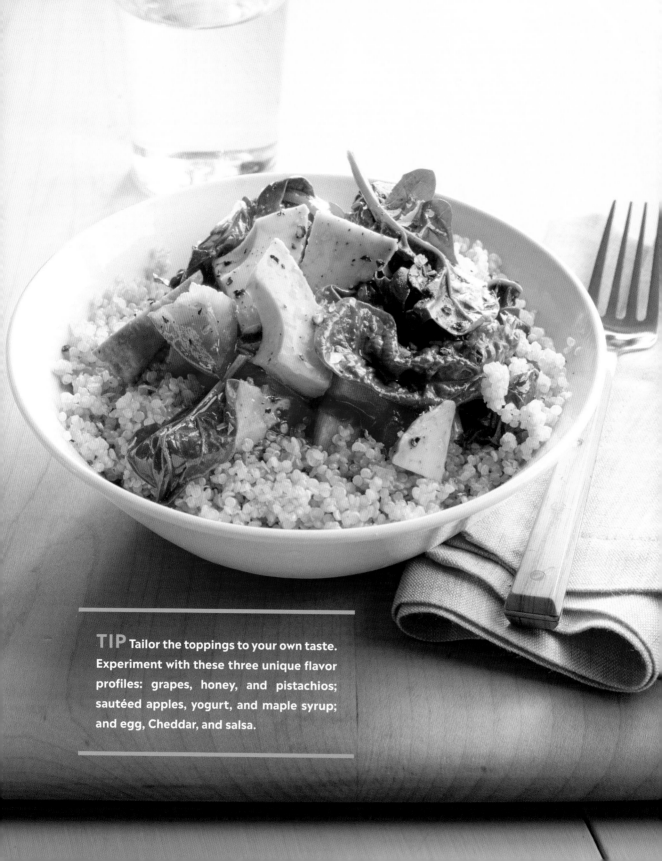

TIP Tailor the toppings to your own taste. Experiment with these three unique flavor profiles: grapes, honey, and pistachios; sautéed apples, yogurt, and maple syrup; and egg, Cheddar, and salsa.

GRAIN BOWL 🌱

Retire your dry cereal and try a new kind of breakfast. Prepared with quinoa, the dish is bursting with protein and healthy fats. Even better, this vegan bowl is entirely customizable, meaning you'll never become bored with it.

1 tablespoon olive oil, plus more for drizzling

1 clove garlic, finely chopped

1 bunch spinach, roughly chopped

¼ teaspoon kosher salt

¼ teaspoon black pepper

2 cups leftover cooked grains (such as farro, brown rice, quinoa, or couscous)

½ avocado, roughly chopped

1 tomato, cut into 1-inch pieces

1. Heat oil in a large nonstick pan on medium. Add garlic and cook until it starts to turn golden brown, 1 minute. Add the spinach, salt, and pepper, tossing just until wilted, 1 to 2 minutes.

2. Divide grains between 2 bowls and top with spinach, avocado, and tomato.

PER SERVING 380 calories, 16 g fat (2.5 g saturated fat), 8 g protein, 305 mg sodium, 54 g carbohydrates, 9 g fiber, 2 g sugars (0 g added sugars), 0 mg cholesterol

STRAWBERRY-THYME MILLET BOWL

TOTAL TIME: 45 MINUTES ◆ SERVES 4

Millet is an ancient whole grain with a consistency somewhere between oatmeal and rice pudding. It has been linked to lower blood sugar and cholesterol levels. Not only that, it's gluten-free and available in most grocery stores.

1 pound strawberries, halved

4 sprigs thyme

1 tablespoon olive oil

1 tablespoon honey

1 cup 2-percent milk, plus more for serving

1 cup millet

1½ teaspoons vanilla extract

2 tablespoons finely chopped pistachios

2 tablespoons hemp seeds

1. Heat oven to 450°F. On a baking sheet, toss strawberries, thyme, oil, and honey. Roast until berries begin to release juices, about 10 minutes. Remove the baking sheet from oven and discard thyme.

2. In a saucepan, bring milk and 1 cup water to a boil. Stir in millet and vanilla, reduce heat to low, cover, and cook until millet is tender and liquid is absorbed, 25 to 30 minutes.

3. Serve millet with berries and pan juices, a splash of milk, pistachios, and hemp seeds.

PER SERVING 355 calories, 10.5 g fat (2 g saturated fat), 11 g protein, 55 mg sodium, 54 g carbohydrates, 7 g fiber, 14 g sugars (4.5 g added sugars), 5 mg cholesterol

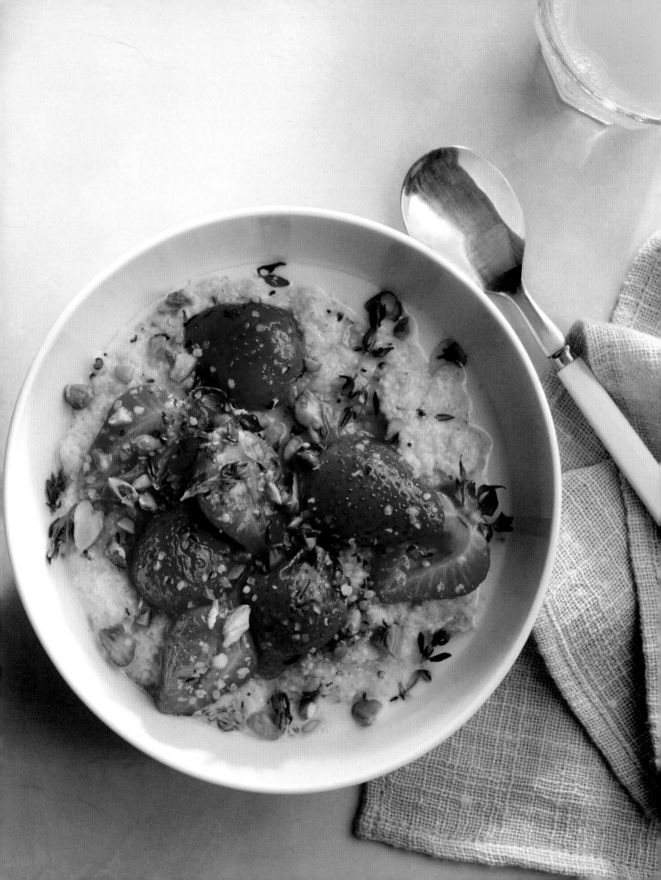

SUNRISE MILLET BOWL

TOTAL TIME: 25 MINUTES ◆ **SERVES 2**

Pomegranate, citrus, and coconut deliver flavor and sweetness, eliminating the need for added sweeteners. Millet's high magnesium content also helps curb cravings for sweets throughout the day.

¾ cup canned light coconut milk, plus more for serving

½ cup millet

¼ teaspoon salt

¼ cup pomegranate seeds

2 tablespoons coconut flakes, toasted

1 grapefruit, peeled and sliced

1 orange, peeled and sliced

2 teaspoons honey, divided

1. In a medium saucepan, combine coconut milk, millet, ¾ cup water, and salt; cook per millet package directions. Divide between 2 bowls, and drizzle each with a bit more coconut milk.

2. Top each serving with pomegranate seeds, coconut flakes, grapefruit, orange, and a teaspoon of honey.

PER SERVING 410 calories, 11 g fat (7.5 g saturated fat), 7 g protein, 160 mg sodium, 72 g carbohydrates, 9 g fiber, 18 g sugars (6 g added sugars), 0 mg cholesterol

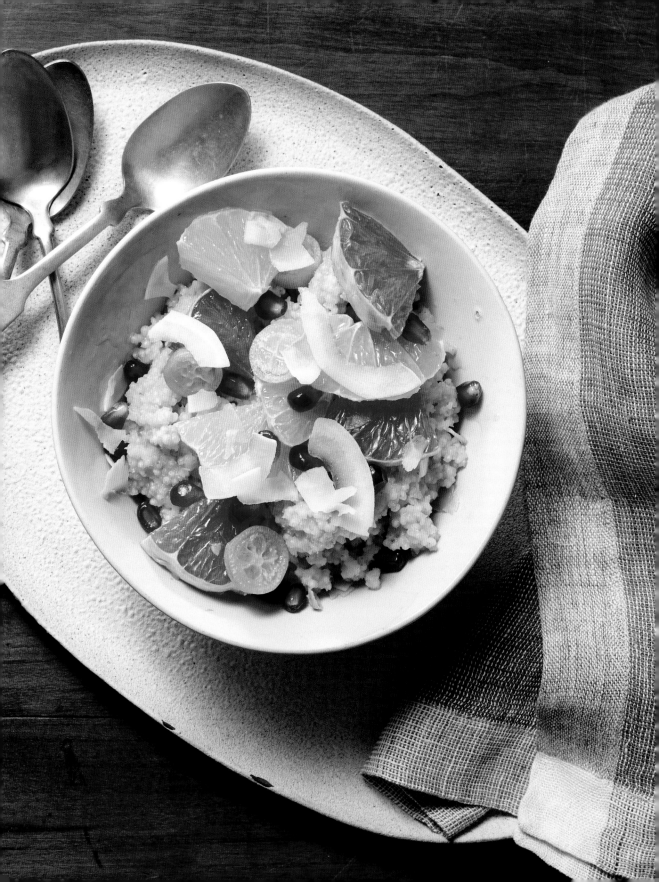

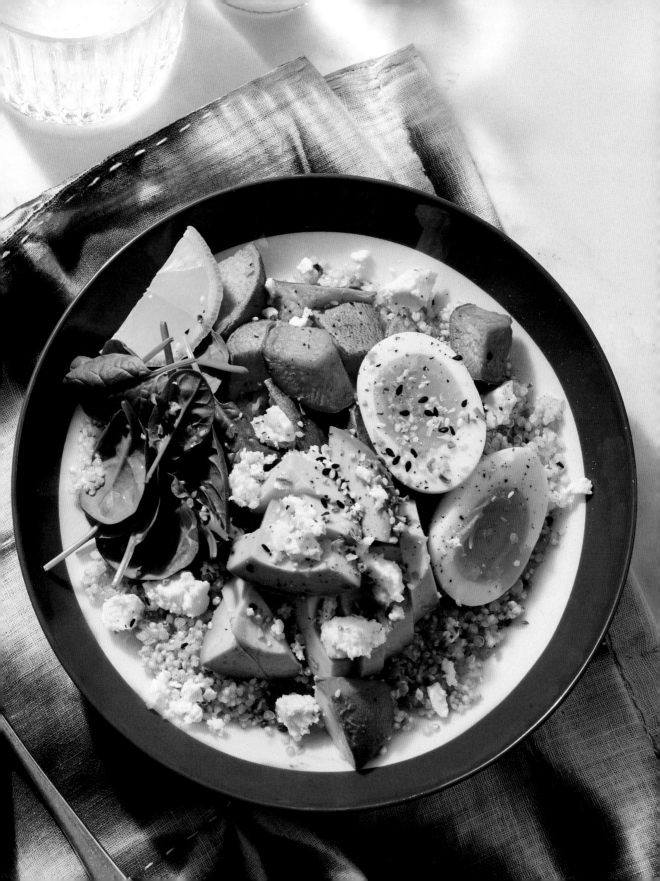

AVOCADO BREAKFAST BOWL

TOTAL TIME: 40 MINUTES ◆ SERVES 4

Sweet potatoes are plant-based superstars: On top of being loaded with vitamins, minerals, and other nutrients, these spuds support healthy vision, boost brain function, and strengthen your immune system.

1 pound sweet potatoes, cut into 1-inch pieces

1 tablespoon olive oil

¼ teaspoon kosher salt

¼ teaspoon black pepper

1 cup quinoa

2 cups baby spinach, roughly chopped

2 small avocados, diced

4 large eggs, soft- or hard-boiled and peeled

Crumbled feta cheese, for topping

Lemon wedges , for serving

Everything-bagel seasoning , for topping

1. Heat oven to 425°F. On a large rimmed baking sheet, toss potatoes with oil, salt, and pepper. Arrange in a single layer and roast until golden brown and tender, about 20 minutes.

2. Meanwhile, cook quinoa per package directions, then fluff with a fork.

3. Divide quinoa among 4 bowls, then top with spinach and potatoes. Add avocado, 1 egg, cheese, and lemon wedge to each serving, and sprinkle with seasoning.

PER SERVING 470 calories, 24 g fat (4 g saturated fat), 16 g protein, 245 mg sodium, 50 g carbohydrates, 12 g fiber, 6 g sugars (0 g added sugars), 186 mg cholesterol

TIP Meal-prepping this dish for throughout the week? Assemble the quinoa and sweet potatoes in storage containers; add spinach in the morning before leaving the house. Keep toppings in a separate container until you're ready to enjoy your healthy breakfast.

BUTTERNUT SQUASH & SPINACH TOASTS

TOTAL TIME: 25 MINUTES ◆ SERVES 4

When you're craving breakfast toast, think beyond avocados. This delicious variation enlists fibrous, nutty butternut squash. One cup of this winter squash provides 100 percent of your daily vitamin A requirement.

1 large butternut squash

1 tablespoon olive oil

2 cloves garlic, chopped

1 bunch spinach, roughly chopped

¼ teaspoon salt

¼ teaspoon black pepper

4 slices bread

⅓ cup grated Gruyère cheese

4 eggs

1. Cut neck off butternut squash; peel and cut into ½-inch pieces.

2. Heat oil in a nonstick skillet. When oil is hot, cook squash, covered, stirring occasionally, 8 minutes. Add garlic, toss, and continue to cook until squash is golden brown and just tender. Toss with spinach and season with salt and pepper.

3. Toast bread and sprinkle each slice with cheese. While topping toast with cooked squash, fry eggs and add 1 to each piece when done.

PER SERVING 265 calories, 14.5 g fat (4 g saturated fat), 13 g protein, 420 mg sodium, 20 g carbohydrates, 3 g fiber, 3 g sugars (1 g added sugars), 194 mg cholesterol

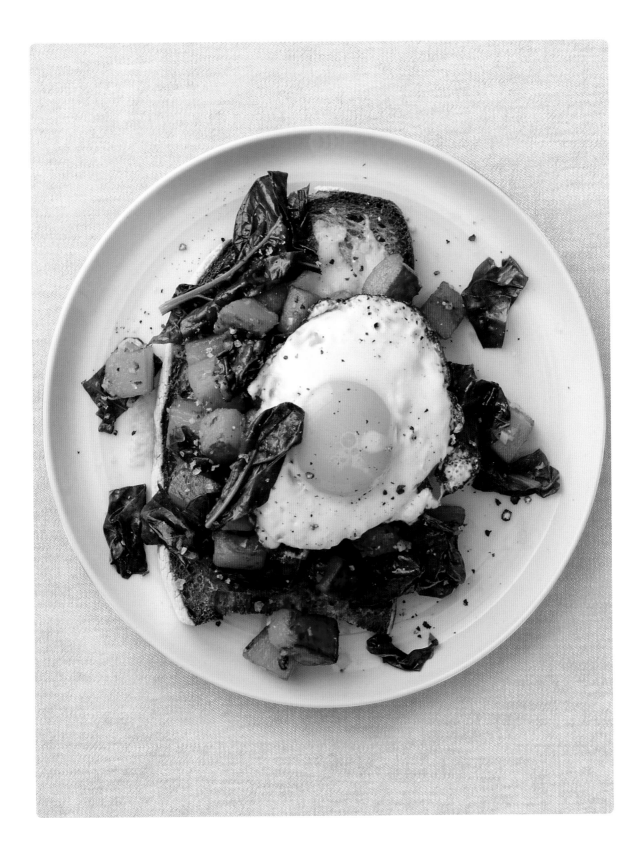

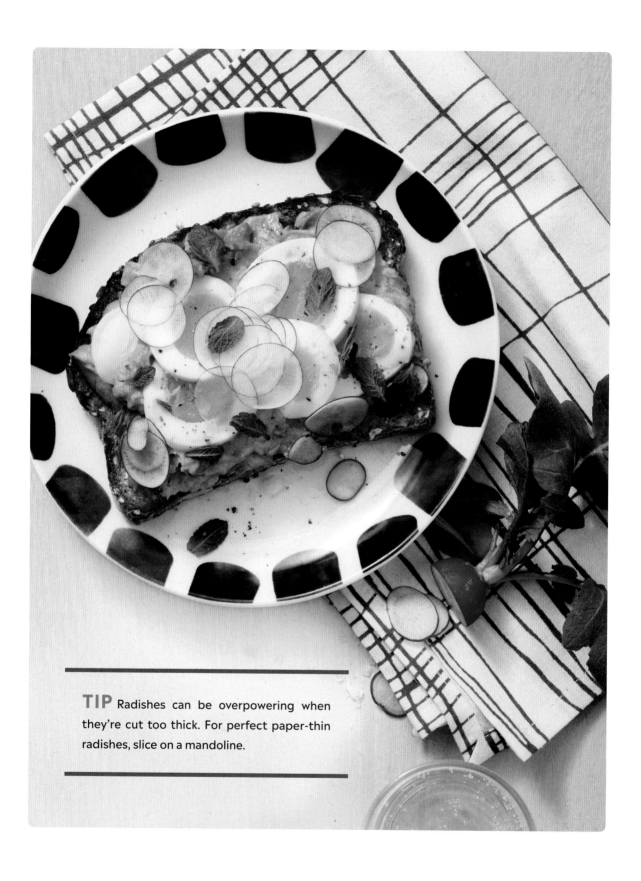

TIP Radishes can be overpowering when they're cut too thick. For perfect paper-thin radishes, slice on a mandoline.

SPRING RADISH & AVOCADO TOAST

TOTAL TIME: 5 MINUTES ◆ SERVES 1

This veggie-forward toast is deliciously light but loaded with healthy fats, potassium, and folates.

1 thin slice whole-grain bread

½ avocado, smashed

Lemon juice

1 hard-boiled egg, thinly sliced

2 small radishes, very thinly sliced

¼ teaspoon salt

¼ teaspoon black pepper

Mint leaves, for topping

1. Toast slice of whole-grain bread.

2. Top with avocado and drizzle with lemon juice. Then top with egg and radishes. Sprinkle with salt, pepper, and mint leaves.

PER SERVING 290 calories, 21 g fat (4 g saturated fat), 12 g protein, 300 mg sodium, 20 g carbohydrates, 9 g fiber, 2.5 g sugars (0 g added sugars), 187 mg cholesterol

NO-BAKE FRUIT & NUT BARS

TOTAL TIME: 45 MINUTES ◆ SERVES 12

Need a nutritious breakfast on the go? These bars are just 215 calories each and can be made up to a month in advance. Store them tightly wrapped in freezer paper in the freezer for maximum freshness.

1 cup pitted Medjool dates

¼ cup nut butter

¼ cup honey

1 teaspoon vanilla extract

1 cup roasted unsalted almonds, roughly chopped

½ cup old-fashioned rolled oats

¾ cup dried fruit (cranberries, golden raisins, sliced apricots)

¼ cup pepitas

1. Line an 8-inch square pan with nonstick foil, leaving some overhang on all sides.

2. In a food processor, chop dates (they will form a ball); transfer to a bowl.

3. In a saucepan, melt nut butter, honey, and vanilla on medium, stirring occasionally to combine, about 1 minute. Add to the bowl; mix to combine.

4. Fold in almonds, oats, fruit, and pepitas. Press into pan and freeze until sliceable, about 30 minutes. Cut into 12 bars. Store in the refrigerator for 14 days or in the freezer for up to a month.

PER SERVING 215 calories, 10.5 g fat (1.5 g saturated fat), 5 g protein, 25 mg sodium, 29 g carbohydrates, 4 g fiber, 22 g sugars (7.5 g added sugars), 0 mg cholesterol

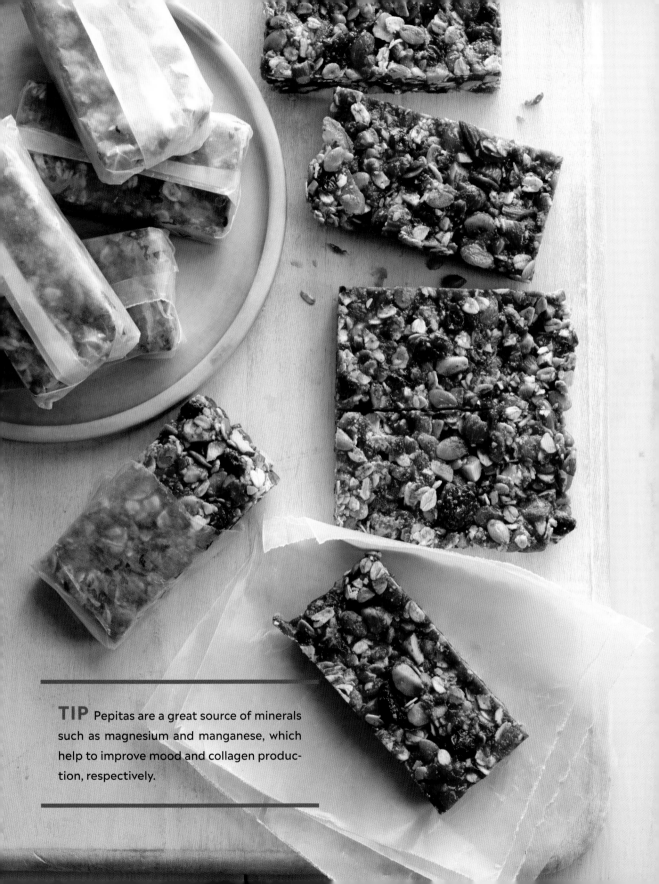

TIP Pepitas are a great source of minerals such as magnesium and manganese, which help to improve mood and collagen production, respectively.

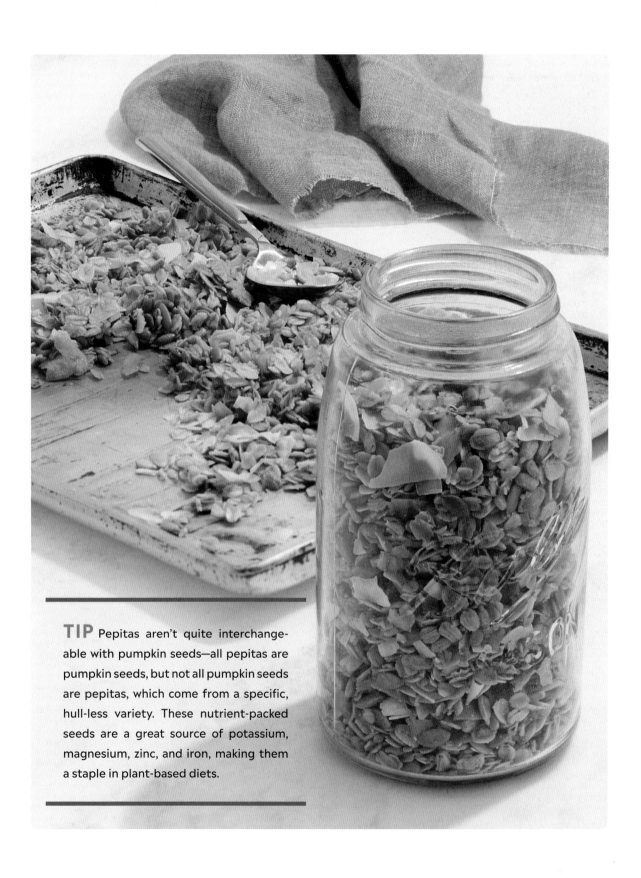

TIP Pepitas aren't quite interchangeable with pumpkin seeds—all pepitas are pumpkin seeds, but not all pumpkin seeds are pepitas, which come from a specific, hull-less variety. These nutrient-packed seeds are a great source of potassium, magnesium, zinc, and iron, making them a staple in plant-based diets.

COCONUT & SEED GRANOLA 🌱

TOTAL TIME: 1 HOUR 15 MINUTES ◆ SERVES 14

Delicious on its own or served with Greek yogurt or your choice of milk, this granola employs pepitas for an earthy, nutty flavor that gets even better when paired with vitamin-B-packed sunflower seeds and manganese-rich coconut.

½ cup olive oil or melted coconut oil

¾ cup pure maple syrup

2 tablespoons turbinado sugar

1 teaspoon kosher salt

3 cups old-fashioned rolled oats

1 cup unsweetened coconut flakes

¾ cup raw sunflower seeds

¾ cup pepitas

1. Heat oven to 300°F. Line a large rimmed baking sheet with parchment paper.

2. In a large bowl, combine oil, maple syrup, sugar, and salt. Add oats, coconut, and seeds. Stir to coat.

3. Spread mixture onto the prepared pan and bake until light golden brown and dry, 45 to 55 minutes, stirring every 15 minutes. Remove from oven and let cool completely.

PER SERVING 300 calories, 19 g fat (5.5 g saturated fat), 6 g protein, 145 mg sodium, 29 g carbohydrates, 4 g fiber, 13.5 g sugars (12.5 g added sugars), 0 mg cholesterol

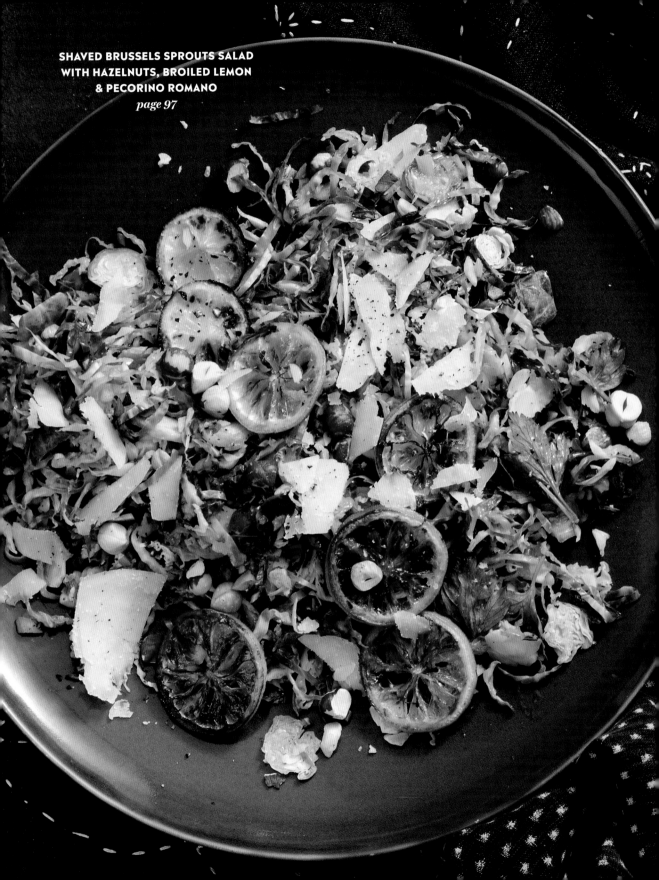

**SHAVED BRUSSELS SPROUTS SALAD
WITH HAZELNUTS, BROILED LEMON
& PECORINO ROMANO**
page 97

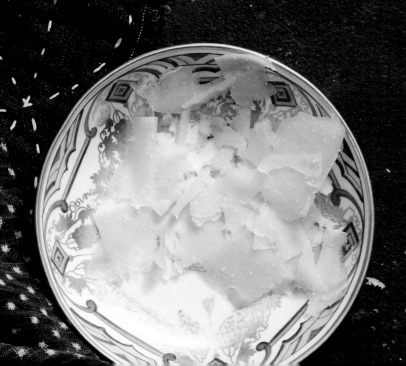

Chapter 2

SOUPS & SALADS

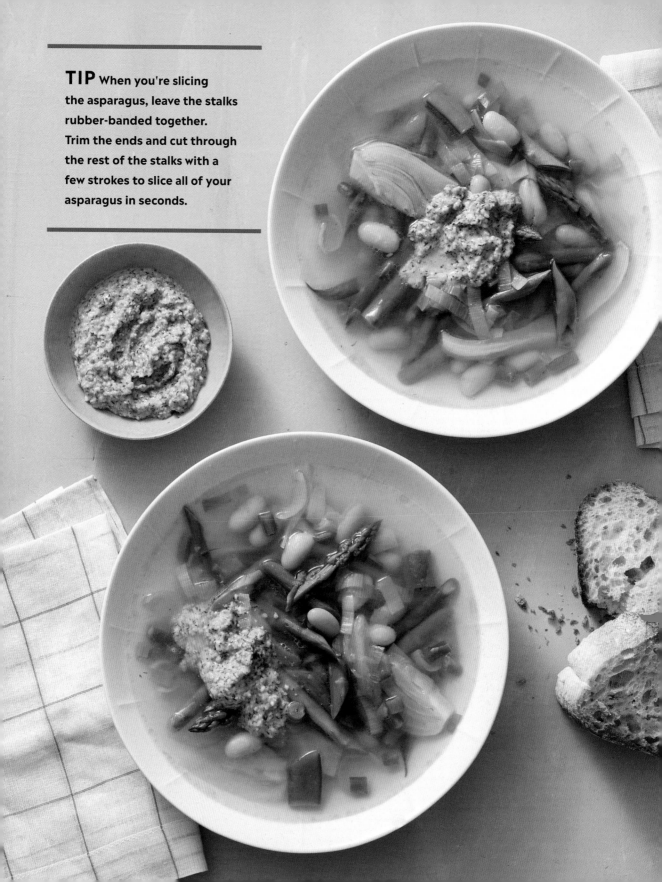

TIP When you're slicing the asparagus, leave the stalks rubber-banded together. Trim the ends and cut through the rest of the stalks with a few strokes to slice all of your asparagus in seconds.

MINESTRONE SOUP

TOTAL TIME: 30 MINUTES ◆ SERVES 4

This colorful spring soup is full of healthy veggies, and the beans offer plant-based protein for a filling meal. Plus, there's an added benefit: Beans have actually been shown to help lower cholesterol.

2 tablespoons olive oil

2 stalks celery, finely chopped

2 leeks, white and light-green parts only, finely chopped

1 onion, finely chopped

¾ teaspoon kosher salt, divided

12 ounces red potatoes, cut into ½-inch pieces

8 sprigs thyme

¼ teaspoon black pepper

1 pound asparagus, trimmed and cut into 1-inch pieces

6 ounces sugar snap peas, halved

1 (15-ounce) can white beans, drained and rinsed

Chopped dill, for topping

Crusty whole-wheat bread, for serving

1. Heat oil in a Dutch oven on medium. Add celery, leeks, onion, and ½ teaspoon salt; cook, covered, stirring occasionally, until tender, 5 to 7 minutes.

2. Add potatoes, thyme, remaining ¼ teaspoon salt, pepper, and 6 cups water. Bring to a boil, then simmer 8 minutes. Add asparagus and simmer 2 minutes.

3. Add sugar snap peas and beans; simmer until vegetables are just tender, 3 to 4 minutes more. Discard thyme. Sprinkle soup with dill and serve with bread, if desired.

PER SERVING 290 calories, 7.5 g fat (1 g saturated fat), 12 g protein, 535 mg sodium, 34 g carbohydrates, 14 g fiber, 7 g sugars (0 g added sugars), 0 mg cholesterol

KALE & CHICKPEA SOUP

TOTAL TIME: 25 MINUTES ◆ SERVES 4

Hearty soups can be made entirely from plant-based ingredients. This one is chock-full of A, B6, and C vitamins from the Tuscan kale plus protein and fiber from the chickpeas. Want to make it vegan? Skip the Pecorino Romano on top.

1 tablespoon olive oil

6 cloves garlic, pressed

1 tablespoon lemon zest

¼ to ½ teaspoon red pepper flakes

½ teaspoon fennel seeds, coarsely crushed

1 (14-ounce) can tomato puree

1 teaspoon salt

1 bunch Tuscan kale, stems and tough ribs discarded, leaves coarsely chopped

1 (15.5-ounce) can chickpeas, drained and rinsed

½ cup grated Pecorino Romano cheese, for topping

Lemon wedges, for serving

1. Heat oil in a large Dutch oven on medium. Add garlic and lemon zest and cook, stirring, 1 minute. Add red pepper flakes and fennel seeds and cook, stirring, 2 minutes more.

2. Add tomato puree, 4 cups water, and salt. Cover and bring to a boil; add kale and simmer 4 minutes.

3. Add chickpeas and simmer until heated through, about 2 minutes more. Top with cheese and serve with lemon wedges.

PER SERVING 335 calories, 10 g fat (4 g saturated fat), 20 g protein, 695 mg sodium, 48 g carbohydrates, 11 g fiber, 8 g sugars (0 g added sugars), 20 mg cholesterol

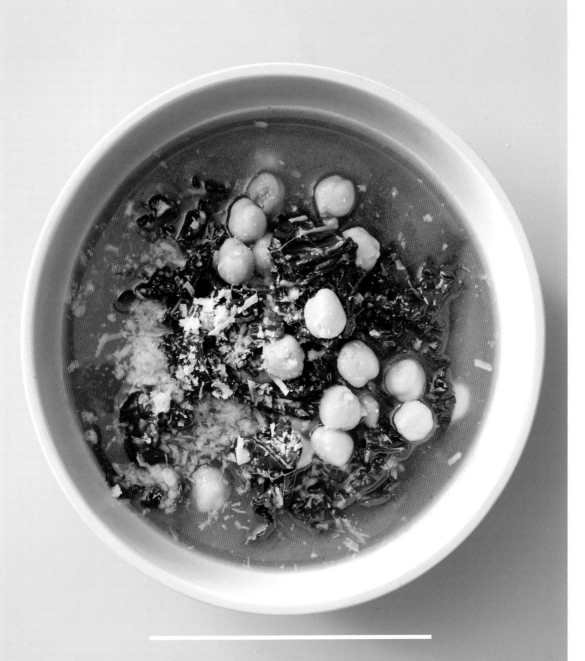

TIP Have leftover cheese rinds? Toss them into the soup while it's simmering for more flavor. Discard them before serving.

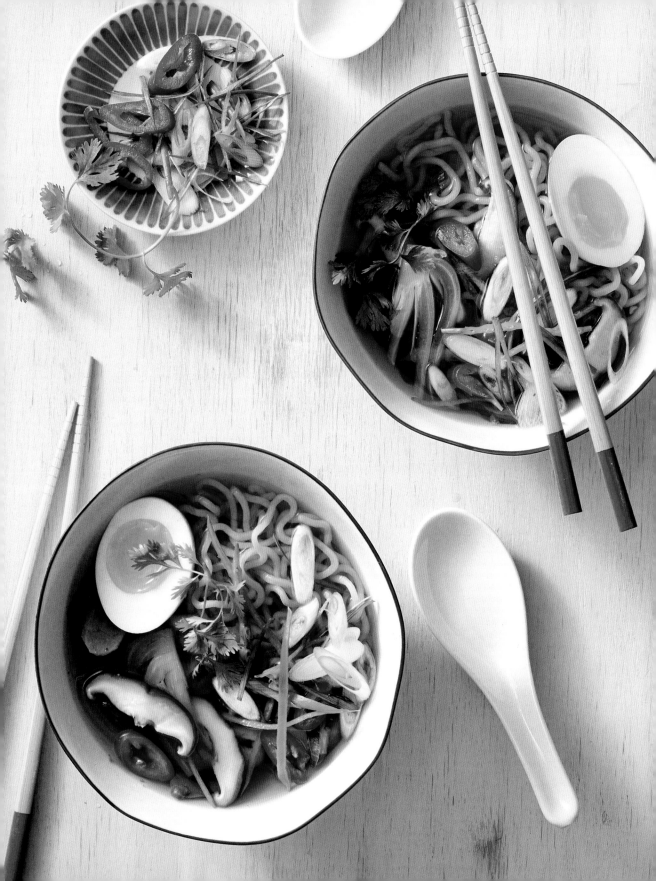

VEGETABLE RAMEN WITH MUSHROOMS & BOK CHOY

TOTAL TIME: 25 MINUTES ◆ SERVES 4

Bok choy is packed with calcium, iron, and vitamins A and C. Combined with mushrooms, snow peas, and the classic soft-boiled eggs, this Japanese noodle soup makes a filling vegetarian dinner.

3 scallions, sliced, white and green parts separated

1 (3-ounce) piece ginger, peeled and very thinly sliced

5 tablespoons low-sodium tamari or soy sauce

6 ounces ramen noodles

6 ounces shiitake mushroom caps, thinly sliced

2 bunches baby bok choy, stems thinly sliced and leaves halved lengthwise

4 ounces snow peas, thinly sliced lengthwise

1 tablespoon rice vinegar

2 soft- or medium-boiled eggs, peeled and halved

½ cup cilantro sprigs, for topping

Thinly sliced red chile, for topping

1. In a large pot, combine scallion whites with ginger and 8 cups water; bring to a boil.

2. Stir in tamari, then add noodles and cook per package directions, adding mushrooms and bok choy 3 minutes after noodles. Remove from heat and stir in snow peas and vinegar.

3. Divide soup among 4 bowls and top each with 1 egg half. Top with scallion greens, cilantro, and chile.

PER SERVING 300 calories, 10 g fat (4.5 g saturated fat), 15 g protein, 1,075 mg sodium, 38 g carbohydrates, 4 g fiber, 4 g sugars (0 g added sugars), 93 mg cholesterol

BUTTERNUT SQUASH & WHITE BEAN SOUP ✿

TOTAL TIME: 45 MINUTES ◆ SERVES 4

Squash is naturally high in potassium—one cup of it has even more than a banana. Potassium helps prevent fatigue, regulates blood pressure, and is essential for muscle and bone health.

1 large butternut squash

2 tablespoons olive oil, divided

1 onion, chopped

2 cloves garlic, finely chopped

1 tablespoon peeled and finely chopped ginger

6 cups low-sodium chicken or vegetable broth

6 sprigs thyme

1 (15-ounce) can white beans, drained and rinsed

1 (15-ounce) can chickpeas, drained and rinsed

½ cup couscous

¼ cup shelled pistachios, roughly chopped

¼ cup cilantro, roughly chopped

¼ cup dried apricots, finely chopped

1 scallion, sliced

1. Cut neck off squash (reserving base for another use), then peel and cut into ½-inch pieces.

2. Heat 1 tablespoon oil in a nonstick skillet on medium. Add squash and cook, covered, stirring occasionally, 8 minutes.

3. Meanwhile, heat remaining 1 tablespoon oil in a Dutch oven on medium. Add onion and cook, covered, stirring occasionally, 6 minutes. Stir in garlic and ginger and cook 1 minute. Add broth, thyme, and cooked squash and bring to a boil.

4. In a medium bowl, use a fork to mash white beans. Add beans to soup along with chickpeas.

5. Cook couscous per package directions; fluff with a fork and fold in pistachios, cilantro, apricots, and scallion. Serve soup topped with couscous mixture.

PER SERVING 560 calories, 14.5 g fat (2 g saturated fat), 26 g protein, 385 mg sodium, 88 g carbohydrates, 19 g fiber, 10 g sugars (0 g added sugars), 0 mg cholesterol

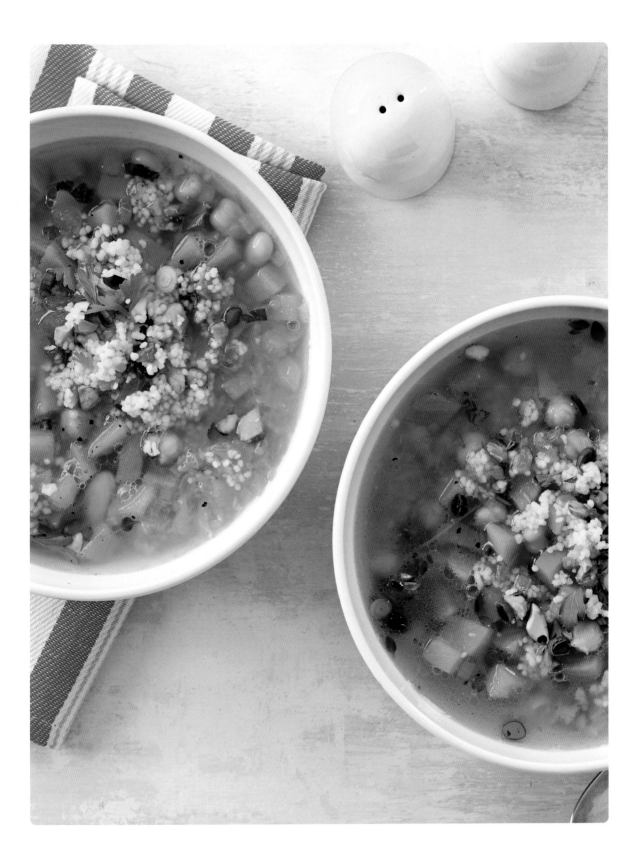

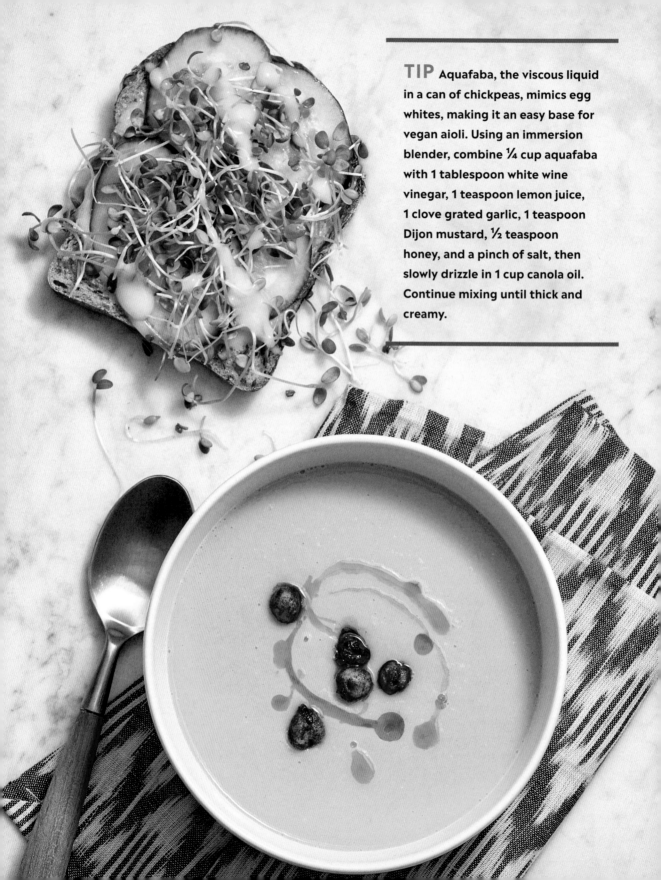

TIP Aquafaba, the viscous liquid in a can of chickpeas, mimics egg whites, making it an easy base for vegan aioli. Using an immersion blender, combine ¼ cup aquafaba with 1 tablespoon white wine vinegar, 1 teaspoon lemon juice, 1 clove grated garlic, 1 teaspoon Dijon mustard, ½ teaspoon honey, and a pinch of salt, then slowly drizzle in 1 cup canola oil. Continue mixing until thick and creamy.

CREAMY CHICKPEA SOUP 🌱

TOTAL TIME: 40 MINUTES ◆ SERVES 4

Whether you call them chickpeas or garbanzo beans, these protein-packed pantry staples deliver a healthy dose of fiber, folate, and iron. Here, they are used as the base of a hearty vegan stew.

1 tablespoon olive oil

1 large onion, thinly sliced

2 large carrots (about 8 ounces), finely chopped

1 leek, white and light-green parts only, sliced

1 clove garlic, sliced

½ teaspoon kosher salt

2 (15-ounce) cans low-sodium chickpeas, drained and rinsed

4 cups low-sodium vegetable broth

¼ cup canola oil

2 teaspoons hot Hungarian paprika

1. Heat olive oil in a large Dutch oven or heavy-bottomed pot on medium. Add onion, carrots, leek, garlic, and salt. Cook, covered, stirring occasionally, 5 minutes.

2. Add all but ¼ cup chickpeas and cook, covered, stirring occasionally, until vegetables are tender, 5 to 6 minutes.

3. Add vegetable broth and 2 cups water; bring to a boil, then reduce to a simmer until vegetables are very soft, 10 to 12 minutes. Remove from heat.

4. While soup simmers, prepare paprika oil: Heat canola oil and paprika in a small saucepan on medium until warm. Remove from heat, strain through a fine-mesh sieve, and let cool. Roughly chop remaining ¼ cup chickpeas.

5. Using an immersion blender or a standard blender, puree soup in batches until very smooth. Serve drizzled with paprika oil and topped with reserved chickpeas. Save remaining paprika oil for another use.

PER SERVING 310 calories, 10.5 g fat (1 g saturated fat), 11 g protein, 555 mg sodium, 45 g carbohydrates, 12 g fiber, 11 g sugars (0 g added sugars), 0 mg cholesterol

SPICED TOMATO SOUP WITH COCONUT FLATBREAD 🌱

TOTAL TIME: 20 MINUTES ◆ SERVES 4

Coconut milk could be a secret weapon in your pantry. It adds a plant-based creamy texture to many soups in place of dairy, plus coconut milk contains MCT fats, which your body uses more rapidly for energy compared to other fats. Coconut flakes are super rich in manganese, a nutrient that stimulates both bone health and metabolism, along with other minerals such as copper, iron, and selenium.

2 tablespoons olive oil, divided

1 large onion, chopped

1 red pepper, chopped

¼ teaspoon salt

2 cloves garlic, finely grated

1 jalapeño, finely grated

1 (1-inch) piece ginger, peeled and finely grated

2 teaspoons ground coriander

1 teaspoon ground cumin

2 pounds tomatoes, roughly chopped

1 (13.5-ounce) can light coconut milk

1 large pocketless pita

2 tablespoons chopped cilantro

2 tablespoons finely shredded coconut

1 tablespoon brown sugar

1. Heat 1 tablespoon oil in a large Dutch oven on medium-low, then add onion, red pepper, and salt; sauté, covered, until tender, 6 minutes.

2. Stir garlic, jalapeño, and ginger into pot with vegetables and cook, 1 minute.

3. Add coriander and cumin; cook, stirring, 1 minute. Add tomatoes, coconut milk, and 2 cups water; bring to a boil, then reduce heat and simmer, 10 minutes.

4. Use a blender to puree soup until smooth.

5. Lightly toast pita. Combine cilantro, coconut, brown sugar, and remaining oil. Spread onto pita and cut into pieces. Serve with soup.

PER SERVING 310 calories, 19 g fat (9 g saturated fat), 6 g protein, 275 mg sodium, 32 g carbohydrates, 6 g fiber, 14.5 g sugars (3.5 g added sugars), 0 mg cholesterol

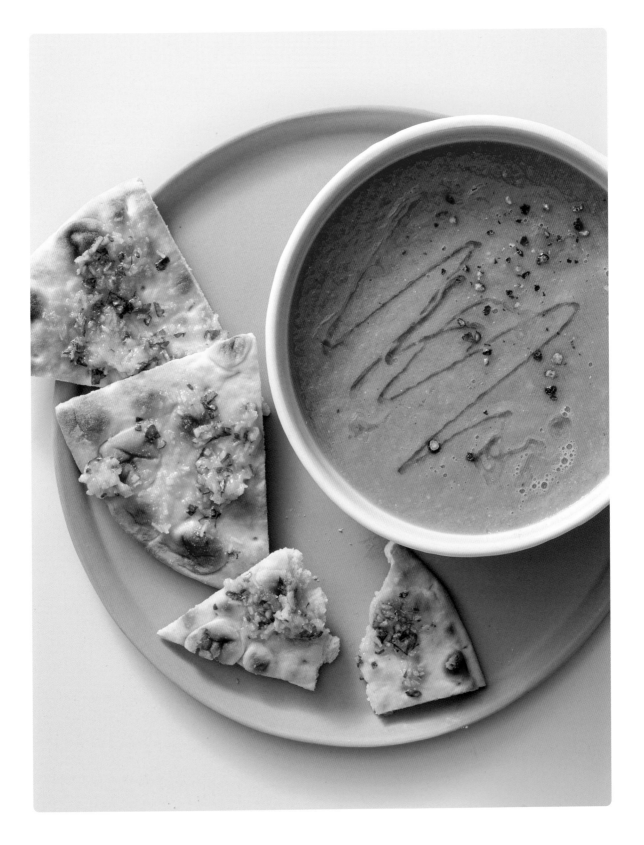

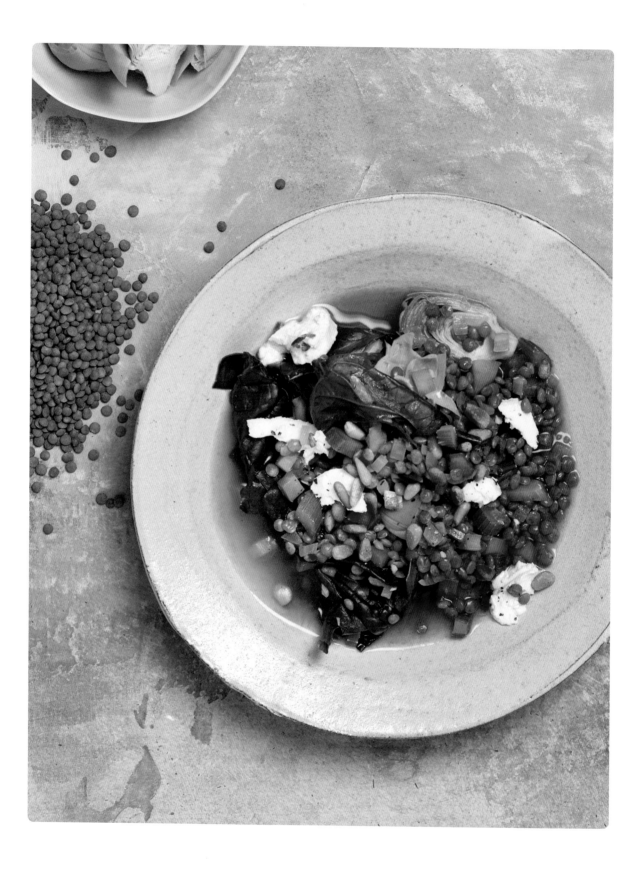

ITALIAN LENTIL STEW

TOTAL TIME: 55 MINUTES ◆ SERVES 4

Lentils are low in calories and packed with minerals and vitamins, making them a nutritional powerhouse—and a particularly tasty one. Small and mighty, lentils are high in fiber, which slows the body's process of turning carbohydrates into glucose, preventing blood sugar spikes and keeping you feeling full.

1 teaspoon olive oil

2 cloves garlic, minced

1 medium carrot, finely chopped

1 stalk celery, finely chopped

1 yellow onion, finely chopped

⅛ teaspoon red pepper flakes

¼ teaspoon salt

2 cups low-sodium vegetable broth

1¼ cups dried lentils

5 cups baby spinach

1 (12-ounce) package frozen artichoke hearts, thawed

2 ounces crumbled goat cheese, for topping

2 tablespoons toasted pine nuts, for topping

1. Heat oil in a saucepan on medium. Add garlic, carrot, celery, onion, red pepper flakes, and salt. Cook, stirring, until onion is translucent, 8 minutes.

2. Stir in broth, lentils, and 3 cups water. Cook until tender, 30 minutes. Add spinach and artichoke hearts; cook 5 minutes more.

3. Divide stew among 4 bowls. Sprinkle with cheese and pine nuts before serving.

PER SERVING 370 calories, 8.5 g fat (2.5 g saturated fat), 22 g protein, 375 mg sodium, 53 g carbohydrates, 26 g fiber, 5 g sugars (0 g added sugars), 18 mg cholesterol

THAI GREEN CURRY SOUP 🌱

TOTAL TIME: 40 MINUTES ◆ SERVES 4

Green curry paste is responsible for giving this soup its bold and delicious flavor. Turmeric, kaffir lime, ginger, chile peppers, and lemongrass all contribute to this unique seasoning—and they also help reduce inflammation, aid digestion, and prevent colds.

1 pound asparagus

4 teaspoons coconut oil, divided

1 small onion, chopped

1 (1-inch) piece ginger, peeled and chopped

1 quart reduced-sodium vegetable broth

1 (13.5-ounce) can light coconut milk

1 tablespoon Thai green curry paste

5 ounces spinach

10 ounces frozen peas, thawed, divided

½ teaspoon kosher salt

½ teaspoon black pepper

1 cup sugar snap peas, trimmed and halved

Mint leaves, for topping

1. Trim asparagus, set stalks aside, and coarsely chop ends.

2. Heat 2 teaspoons oil in a pot on medium. Add onion, ginger, and asparagus ends. Cook until veggies soften, 5 minutes.

3. Add broth, coconut milk, and curry paste. Boil, reduce to simmer, and cook until veggies are tender, 8 minutes. Add spinach and 5 ounces thawed peas; cook until spinach wilts.

4. Remove from heat. With an immersion blender or a standard blender, puree soup in batches until very smooth; season with salt and pepper, or to taste.

5. Cut asparagus stalks into 1-inch pieces. Heat remaining 2 teaspoons oil in a skillet on medium-high. Add stalks, sugar snap peas, and remaining peas. Sauté until crisp-tender, 3 minutes. Serve soup topped with veggies and mint.

PER SERVING 260 calories, 11.5 g fat (9 g saturated fat), 10 g protein, 610 mg sodium, 29 g carbohydrates, 9 g fiber, 11 g sugars (0 g added sugars), 0 mg cholesterol

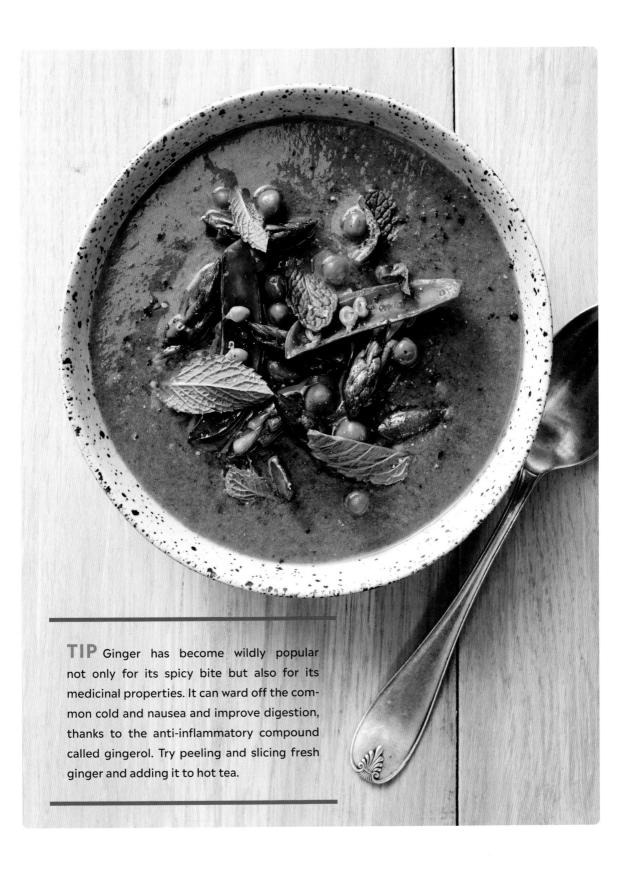

TIP Ginger has become wildly popular not only for its spicy bite but also for its medicinal properties. It can ward off the common cold and nausea and improve digestion, thanks to the anti-inflammatory compound called gingerol. Try peeling and slicing fresh ginger and adding it to hot tea.

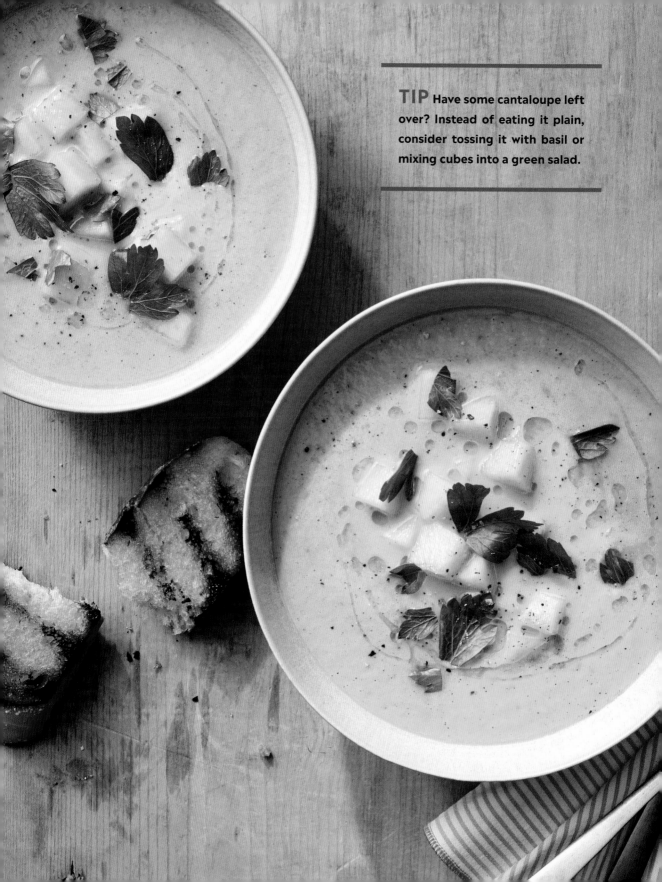

TIP Have some cantaloupe left over? Instead of eating it plain, consider tossing it with basil or mixing cubes into a green salad.

CANTALOUPE GAZPACHO 🌱

Like carrots, cantaloupe is rich in beta-carotene, a powerful antioxidant that helps keep skin healthy and boosts immunity. You've never tasted cantaloupe like this before.

8 slices whole-wheat baguette

4 tablespoons extra virgin olive oil, divided, plus more for topping

1 small jalapeño

1 yellow pepper

½ small white onion, roughly chopped

4 cups cantaloupe chunks, plus 1½ cups diced for serving

3 tablespoons sherry vinegar

2 cloves garlic

1 teaspoon kosher salt

½ teaspoon black pepper

Parsley leaves, for topping

1. Heat grill (or grill pan) on medium. Brush bread slices with 2 tablespoons oil and grill until toasted, flipping once, 3 to 5 minutes. Place 2 pieces in a blender.

2. Increase heat to medium-high. Grill peppers, turning until charred but still crisp, 10 minutes; grill onion until tender, flipping once, 8 minutes.

3. When cool enough to handle, remove seeds and stems from peppers and add to blender along with onion, 4 cups cantaloupe chunks, ⅓ cup water, vinegar, garlic, salt, black pepper, and remaining 2 tablespoons oil. Blend until smooth, then refrigerate to chill.

4. Top bowls of chilled soup with remaining diced cantaloupe, parsley, and a drizzle of olive oil. Serve with remaining bread.

PER SERVING 220 calories, 11 g fat (1.5 g saturated fat), 4 g protein, 485 mg sodium, 27 g carbohydrates, 3 g fiber, 12 g sugars (1 g added sugars), 0 mg cholesterol

CURRIED CARROT-LENTIL SOUP 🌱

This soup is a guilt-free, low-calorie comfort food. Fragrant curry powder helps ease digestion and might even boost your immune system.

1 tablespoon olive oil

1 medium onion, chopped

2 teaspoons curry powder

½ teaspoon turmeric

¼ teaspoon cayenne

1¼ cups (8 ounces) dried red lentils, picked over

¾ pound (about 5 medium) carrots, cut into ½-inch rounds

2 tablespoons lime juice

¼ cup chopped cilantro leaves, plus sprigs for garnish

Kosher salt

Black pepper

1. Heat oil in a large saucepan on medium. Add onion and cook, stirring, until softened, about 4 minutes. Stir in curry powder, turmeric, and cayenne; cook, stirring, 1 minute more.

2. Add lentils and 6 cups water. Bring to a boil. Skim to remove foam; simmer lentils, partially covered, 20 minutes. Add carrots and simmer, partially covered, until tender, about 15 minutes more.

3. Puree soup in blender, working in batches, and return to the saucepan.

4. Warm soup on medium heat, stirring, until heated through. Stir in lime juice and chopped cilantro. Season with salt and pepper to taste. Add additional water if soup is too thick. Ladle into bowls and garnish with cilantro sprigs.

PER SERVING 285 calories, 4 g fat (0.5 g saturated fat), 16 g protein, 75 mg sodium, 46 g carbohydrates, 6 g fiber, 8.5 g sugars (0 g added sugars), 0 mg cholesterol

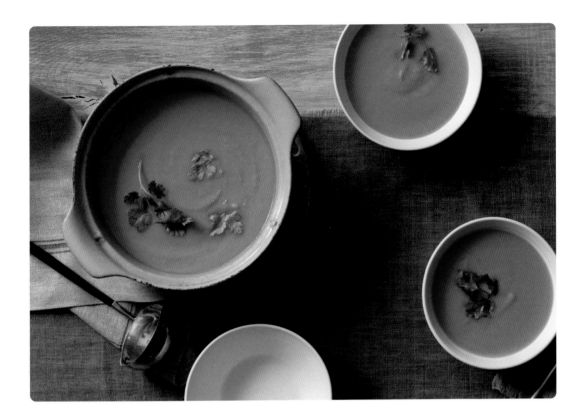

3 HEALTH BENEFITS *of* TURMERIC

Grown throughout India and other parts of Asia, turmeric is a staple of Ayurvedic medicine. Today, it's mainly found in spice or supplement form and commonly used to brighten up curries, stir-fries, soups, and even smoothies. Here are a few more reasons why turmeric deserves a spot on your spice rack.

Turmeric may help improve your memory. *The American Journal of Geriatric Psychiatry* reported that a March 2018 study of people aged 51 to 84 found that those who took a 90-milligram curcumin supplement twice a day for 18 months saw a boost in memory compared with those who took a placebo. The study was small and more research will be needed to confirm these findings, but some scientists believe that curcumin's anti-inflammatory effects might protect the brain from memory-related diseases such as Alzheimer's.

Turmeric might ward off heart disease. Curcumin's antioxidants and anti-inflammatory compounds may help protect against certain heart conditions, including diabetic cardiomyopathy (heart muscle disease), arrhythmia (irregular heartbeat), and more, according to a 2017 review in the journal *Pharmacological Research*.

Turmeric can help ease osteoarthritis pain. Osteoarthritis is the most common cause of disability in the United States. A 2016 research review found that taking curcumin for four weeks, however, could help relieve osteoarthritis pain in people who already have the condition—an effect that's comparable to taking NSAIDs or glucosamine.

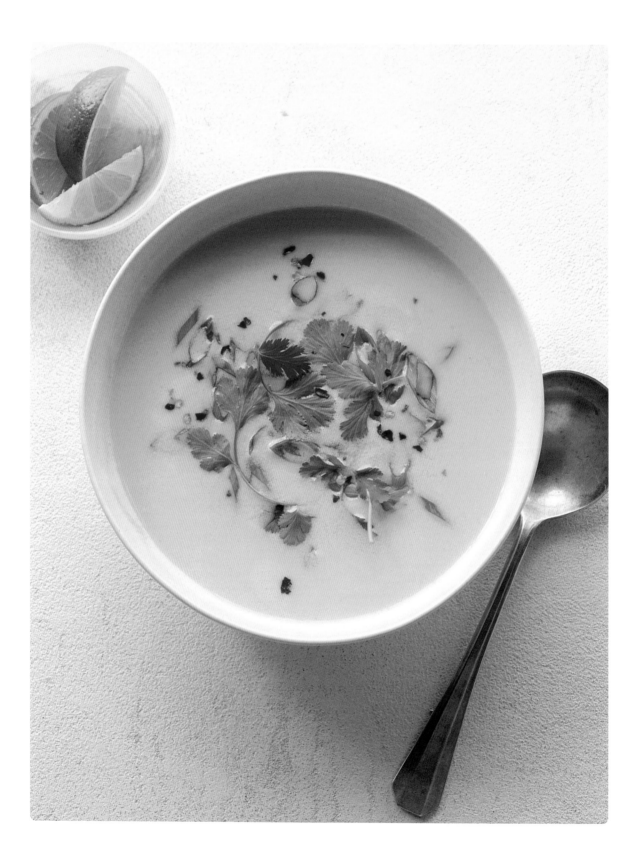

CORN & COCONUT SOUP

TOTAL TIME: 15 MINUTES ◆ SERVES 4

This sweet and creamy soup is just about the definition of simple—all you need to do is prep these easy-to-find and nutrient-rich ingredients, puree, and serve.

1½ cups corn kernels

1 (13.5-ounce) can light coconut milk

1 lime, juiced, plus wedges for serving

2 teaspoons fish sauce

½ teaspoon red pepper flakes, plus more for topping

2 scallions, sliced, white and green parts separated

⅛ teaspoon kosher salt

½ cup cilantro

1. In a blender, combine corn, coconut milk, lime juice, fish sauce, red pepper flakes, scallion whites, and salt.

2. Puree until smooth. Strain, and discard solids. Top with cilantro, red pepper flakes, scallion greens, and serve with lime wedges.

PER SERVING 155 calories, 8.5 g fat (5 g saturated fat), 5 g protein, 325 mg sodium, 19 g carbohydrates, 2 g fiber, 6 g sugars (0 g added sugars), 0 mg cholesterol

ARUGULA SALAD WITH ZUCCHINI RIBBONS

TOTAL TIME: 15 MINUTES ◆ SERVES 4

This vitamin-C-packed dish is appetizing as is, but it's also easily customizable. Add a boost of protein with your favorite plant-based variety or grilled chicken.

1 cup arugula

1 small zucchini (or ½ large)

⅔ cup pecan halves (about 2 ounces)

⅓ cup roasted salted sunflower seeds

1 ounce Parmesan cheese, shaved

1 lemon, halved

2 tablespoons orange zest

¼ cup extra virgin olive oil

1. Place arugula in a large bowl. Using vegetable peeler, shave zucchini to make ribbons. Top arugula with zucchini ribbons.

2. Sprinkle greens with pecans, sunflower seeds, and cheese. Squeeze lemon over salad. Sprinkle with orange zest and drizzle with oil. Serve immediately.

PER SERVING 330 calories, 32 g fat (5 g saturated fat), 7 g protein, 155 mg sodium, 7 g carbohydrates, 3 g fiber, 2 g sugars (0 g added sugars), 6 mg cholesterol

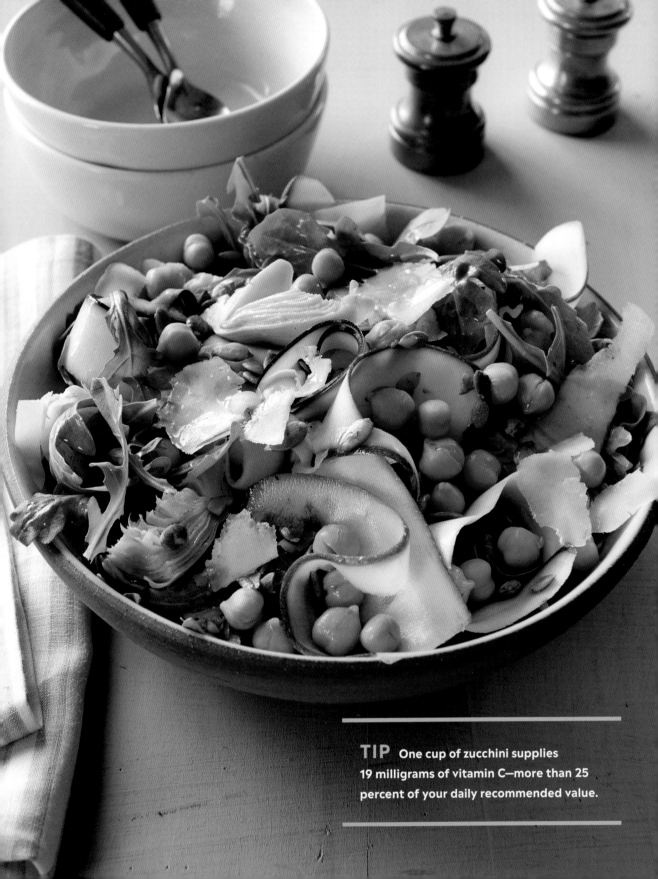

TIP One cup of zucchini supplies 19 milligrams of vitamin C—more than 25 percent of your daily recommended value.

NIÇOISE SALAD WITH SALMON

TOTAL TIME: 20 MINUTES ◆ SERVES 3

Easing into the plant-based plan? This summery salad has the perfect ratio of animal products to veggies: Plants take up about three-quarters of the plate. And if you plan to eat an animal protein, heart-healthy salmon is a great choice. Want to make it entirely plant-based? Sub beans or legumes of your choice.

6 small red potatoes, quartered

Salt

½ pound green beans

2 cups spinach, chopped

¼ cup basil

3 hard-boiled eggs, peeled and quartered

1 (4-ounce) can wild salmon, drained

1 medium tomato, cut into bite-size wedges

½ cup kalamata olives

Homemade vinaigrette (such as the Dijon vinaigrette on page 98), for topping

1. In a small bowl covered with a lid or waxed paper, microwave potatoes until fork-tender, 5 to 7 minutes. Sprinkle with salt to taste.

2. In a small pot of boiling water, blanch green beans, 2 to 3 minutes. Drain and plunge into ice water.

3. Divide spinach and basil among 3 plates, then evenly top with potatoes, green beans, eggs, salmon, tomato, and olives, arranging each ingredient in a small section. Dress with your favorite homemade vinaigrette.

PER SERVING 450 calories, 13 g fat (3 g saturated fat), 22 g protein, 730 mg sodium, 66 g carbohydrates, 9 g fiber, 9 g sugars (0 g added sugars), 214 mg cholesterol

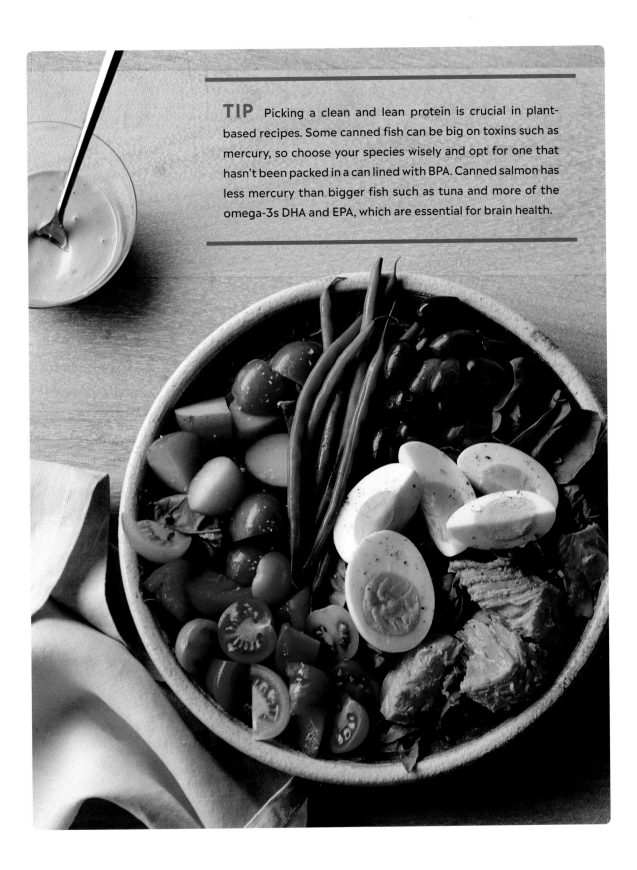

TIP Picking a clean and lean protein is crucial in plant-based recipes. Some canned fish can be big on toxins such as mercury, so choose your species wisely and opt for one that hasn't been packed in a can lined with BPA. Canned salmon has less mercury than bigger fish such as tuna and more of the omega-3s DHA and EPA, which are essential for brain health.

TOMATO-NECTARINE CARPACCIO 🌱

TOTAL TIME: 5 MINUTES   ◆   SERVES 4

Carpaccio is traditionally a dish of meat or fish thinly sliced and served as an appetizer. This vegan spin with summer fruits offers plenty of fiber, potassium, and vitamins A and C.

2 heirloom tomatoes, thinly sliced

1 nectarine, thinly sliced

4 teaspoons olive oil

4 teaspoons champagne vinegar

¼ teaspoon flaked salt

Basil leaves, for topping

Mint leaves, for topping

On a platter, arrange tomato and nectarine slices. Drizzle with oil and vinegar, then sprinkle with salt and a handful of mixed small basil and mint leaves.

PER SERVING 65 calories, 5 g fat (0.5 g saturated fat), 1 g protein, 150 mg sodium, 7 g carbohydrates, 1 g fiber, 4.5 g sugars (0 g added sugars), 0 mg cholesterol

TIP Heirloom tomatoes vary in size and color. They feature a deeper, sweeter taste than non-heirloom varieties and are available in the summer months. Although often priced higher than other tomatoes, heirloom tomatoes have a similar nutritional content, so if they are not available, you can sub another variety.

90   THE PLANT-BASED PLAN

SOUTHWESTERN CHOPPED SALAD

TOTAL TIME: 20 MINUTES ◆ SERVES 4

Cilantro-lime dressing steals the show in this bold salad, which comes in at an almost unbelievable 295 calories per serving, along with lots of protein and fiber. Want more green goodness? Dice your extra avocado half and toss it in.

½ avocado

2 tablespoons plain fat-free Greek yogurt

½ cup cilantro

¼ cup lime juice

1 head romaine lettuce, chopped

1 (15-ounce) can low-sodium black beans, drained and rinsed

1 cucumber, sliced

1 red pepper, sliced

Corn tortillas, sliced

1. Heat oven to 425°F. In a blender, puree avocado, yogurt, cilantro, lime juice, and ¼ cup water.

2. Toss dressing with romaine lettuce. Fold in black beans, cucumber, and red pepper.

3. Place sliced tortillas on a baking sheet and bake until crisp, about 4 to 5 minutes.

4. Top salad with tortilla strips before serving.

PER SERVING 245 calories, 5 g fat (1 g saturated fat), 12 g protein, 130 mg sodium, 42 g carbohydrates, 15 g fiber, 5 g sugars (0 g added sugars), 0 mg cholesterol

TIP For more protein, add 1 pound cooked shrimp to this dish. When shopping, look for wild-caught shrimp, which are largely free of antibiotics and hormones.

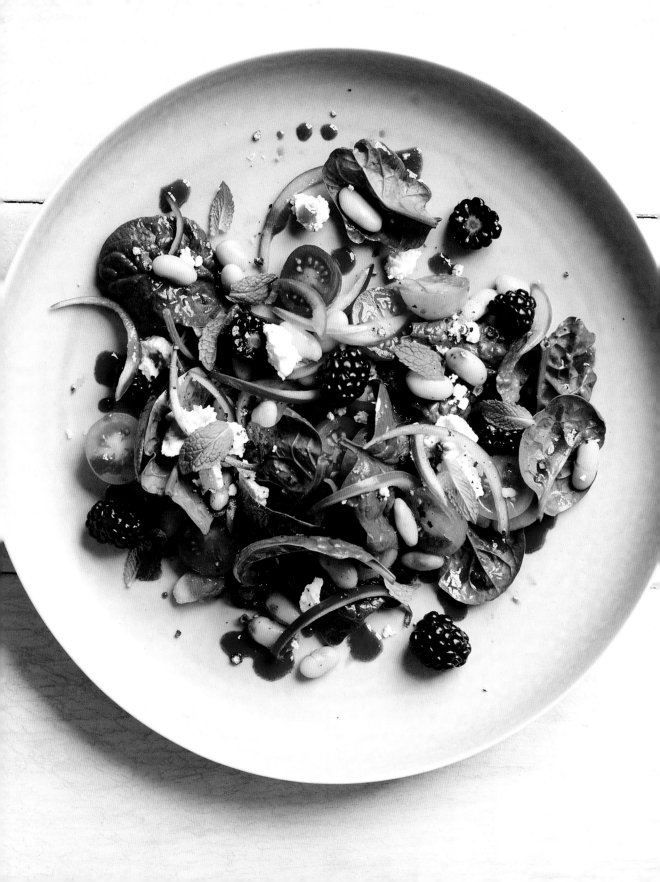

SPINACH SALAD WITH WARM BLACKBERRY VINAIGRETTE

TOTAL TIME: 25 MINUTES ◆ SERVES 4

Feeling run down? The combo of spinach and blackberries in this salad provides you with a good source of riboflavin and B vitamins that alert the immune system to fight infection.

1½ cups blackberries, divided

¼ cup balsamic or red wine vinegar

2 tablespoons olive oil

1 teaspoon Dijon mustard

Kosher salt

Black pepper

1 (10-ounce) package baby spinach

1 (15.5-ounce) can cannellini beans, drained and rinsed

1 cup cherry tomatoes in different colors, halved

¼ small red onion, thinly sliced

2 tablespoons herbs (such as mint, basil, and parsley), coarsely chopped

¼ cup crumbled feta cheese, for topping

1. In a blender, puree 1 cup berries with ¼ cup water until smooth. Strain through a fine-mesh sieve into a small saucepan.

2. Add vinegar and oil; whisk to combine. Whisk in mustard and a pinch each salt and pepper, then cook on medium heat, whisking occasionally, until warm.

3. In a large bowl, toss spinach with warm dressing to coat. Add beans, tomatoes, onion, and herbs, and toss to combine. Serve topped with cheese and remaining ½ cup berries.

PER SERVING 225 calories, 9.5 g fat (2.5 g saturated fat), 8 g protein, 465 mg sodium, 29 g carbohydrates, 10 g fiber, 7 g sugars (0 g added sugars), 8 mg cholesterol

CORN, MANGO & EDAMAME SALAD 🌱

TOTAL TIME: 15 MINUTES ♦ SERVES 6

In addition to folate and fiber, corn contains a carotenoid called beta-cryptoxanthin. Eating a diet high in this compound, which is also found in papaya, pumpkin, and tangerines, may reduce the risk of lung cancer.

2 cups frozen shelled edamame

1½ cups corn kernels

1½ cups mango cubes

1 cup chopped tomato

½ cup chopped red onion

2 tablespoons chopped cilantro

1 tablespoon extra virgin olive oil

1 tablespoon lime juice

¾ teaspoon salt

¼ teaspoon ground black pepper

1. Prepare edamame per package directions. Drain and rinse under cold water.

2. Transfer to a large bowl. Stir in corn, mango, tomato, onion, cilantro, oil, lime juice, salt, and pepper. Toss well.

PER SERVING 160 calories, 5 g fat (0.5 g saturated fat), 9 g protein, 305 mg sodium, 22 g carbohydrates, 6 g fiber, 10 g sugars (0 g added sugars), 0 mg cholesterol

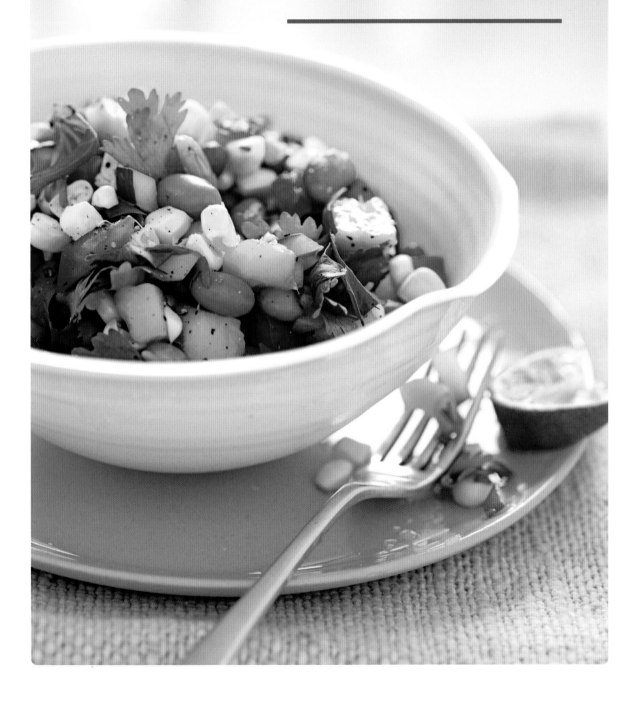

TIP One serving of this salad supplies more than 20 percent of your daily fiber needs—so go ahead, take a second helping!

SQUASH & WATERCRESS SALAD WITH COFFEE VINAIGRETTE

TOTAL TIME: 45 MINUTES ◆ SERVES 2

To conquer the midday slump, whip up this salad, which combines the gut-friendly nutrients of squash and the mood-boosting goodness of watercress.

4 cups diced kabocha squash

2 cloves garlic, smashed

1 tablespoon olive oil

½ teaspoon salt, divided

½ teaspoon black pepper, divided

2½ cups watercress

2 hard-boiled eggs, halved

1 tablespoon brewed hot coffee

1 tablespoon sugar

1 teaspoon sherry vinegar

2 tablespoons grapeseed oil

2 teaspoons sunflower seeds, for topping

1. Heat oven to 400°F. On a rimmed baking sheet, toss squash with garlic, olive oil, and ¼ teaspoon each salt and pepper. Roast until tender, 30 to 35 minutes.

2. In a bowl, mix cooked squash with watercress and hard-boiled eggs.

3. Make the dressing: Whisk together coffee and sugar until dissolved. Whisk in sherry vinegar, grapeseed oil, and remaining ¼ teaspoon each salt and pepper.

4. Sprinkle sunflower seeds over salad and drizzle with vinaigrette.

PER SERVING 370 calories, 17 g fat (3 g saturated fat), 11 g protein, 560 mg sodium, 47 g carbohydrates, 3 g fiber, 15 g sugars (6 g added sugars), 187 mg cholesterol

TIP Watercress belongs to the cruciferous family of vegetables, which also includes kale, arugula, and broccoli. The entire family is rich in folate, vitamin K, and fiber, making them some of the healthiest greens around.

SHAVED BRUSSELS SPROUTS SALAD WITH HAZELNUTS, BROILED LEMON & PECORINO ROMANO

TOTAL TIME: 25 MINUTES ◆ SERVES 8

Brussels sprouts are nutritional superstars on their own, thanks to glucosinolates—compounds linked to lowering cancer risk. With crunchy nuts and sharp cheese, this dish is a hearty vegetable-forward side or main. See the photo on page 62.

½ cup hazelnuts

1½ pounds Brussels sprouts, trimmed

1 lemon, halved crosswise

1 teaspoon plus 3 tablespoons olive oil

¾ teaspoon kosher salt

¼ teaspoon black pepper

3 tablespoons finely chopped chives

½ cup flat-leaf parsley leaves

4 ounces Pecorino Romano cheese, shaved

1. Heat oven to 325°F. Arrange hazelnuts on a rimmed baking sheet; roast until deep golden brown, 10 to 15 minutes. Transfer to a clean dish towel. When cool, rub in towel to remove skins, then coarsely chop nuts and set aside.

2. Using a food processor fitted with the thinnest slicing blade, thinly slice Brussels sprouts, yielding about 6 cups. Alternatively, you can thinly slice with a chef's knife.

3. Heat broiler. Line the same rimmed baking sheet with nonstick foil. Cut half the lemon into ⅓-inch slices, arrange on the baking sheet, and brush with 1 teaspoon oil. Broil until charred and tender, 2 to 3 minutes. Let cool, then chop, if desired; transfer to a large bowl.

4. Into the large bowl, juice remaining lemon half, then add remaining 3 tablespoons oil, salt, and pepper. Add Brussels sprouts and toss to coat; fold in chives, parsley, and half the cheese and nuts. Arrange on a platter; top with remaining cheese and nuts.

PER SERVING 195 calories, 14.5 g fat (3.5 g saturated fat), 9 g protein, 370 mg sodium, 9 g carbohydrates, 4 g fiber, 2 g sugars (0 g added sugars), 15 mg cholesterol

BLUEBERRY-ARUGULA SALAD WITH DIJON VINAIGRETTE

TOTAL TIME: 15 MINUTES ◆ SERVES 4

Skip store-bought dressings whenever possible—they often have hidden added sugars. Homemade dressings allow you to control the ingredients, are easy to make, and taste fresher.

2 tablespoons extra virgin olive oil

2 tablespoons lemon juice

1 teaspoon Dijon mustard

1 teaspoon honey

1 clove garlic, minced

¼ teaspoon salt

¼ teaspoon black pepper

8 cups arugula

⅓ cup coarsely chopped almonds

¾ cup blueberries

2 ounces crumbled herbed goat cheese

1. Make the vinaigrette. In a jar, combine oil, lemon juice, mustard, honey, garlic, salt, and pepper. Cap and shake until combined.

2. In a large bowl, toss arugula with almonds. Add blueberries and cheese. Drizzle with vinaigrette and serve.

PER SERVING 205 calories, 17 g fat (3.5 g saturated fat), 6 g protein, 130 mg sodium, 11 g carbohydrates, 3 g fiber, 6 g sugars (1 g added sugars), 15 mg cholesterol

TIP This salad is packed with plant-based nutrients. The arugula serves up calcium and potassium, while the blueberries contain fiber, magnesium, and potassium, as well. Almonds are a good source of healthy fat.

QUINOA, BLACK BEAN & AVOCADO SALAD

TOTAL TIME: 30 MINUTES ◆ **SERVES 4**

The key to a harmonious grain-based salad is the right mix of veggies and starches. The high fiber content in quinoa and black beans will satisfy your hunger, while the creamy avocado delivers a welcome dose of healthy fats.

2½ cups precooked quinoa

1 (10-ounce) can black beans, drained and rinsed

1 cup grape tomatoes, halved

½ avocado, chopped

1 cup cilantro leaves

¼ cup lime juice

2 tablespoons extra virgin olive oil

½ teaspoon lime zest

1 clove garlic

½ teaspoon black pepper

¼ teaspoon salt

1. In a bowl, combine quinoa, black beans, grape tomatoes, and avocado.

2. In a food processor, pulse cilantro, lime juice, oil, lime zest, garlic, pepper, and salt. Toss with quinoa blend and chill for 15 minutes before serving.

PER SERVING 335 calories, 13 g fat (2 g saturated fat), 11 g protein, 485 mg sodium, 44 g carbs, 10 g fiber, 2.5 g sugars (0 g added sugars), 0 mg cholesterol

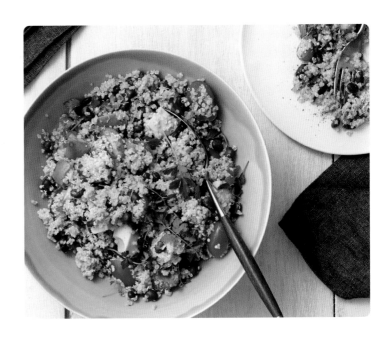

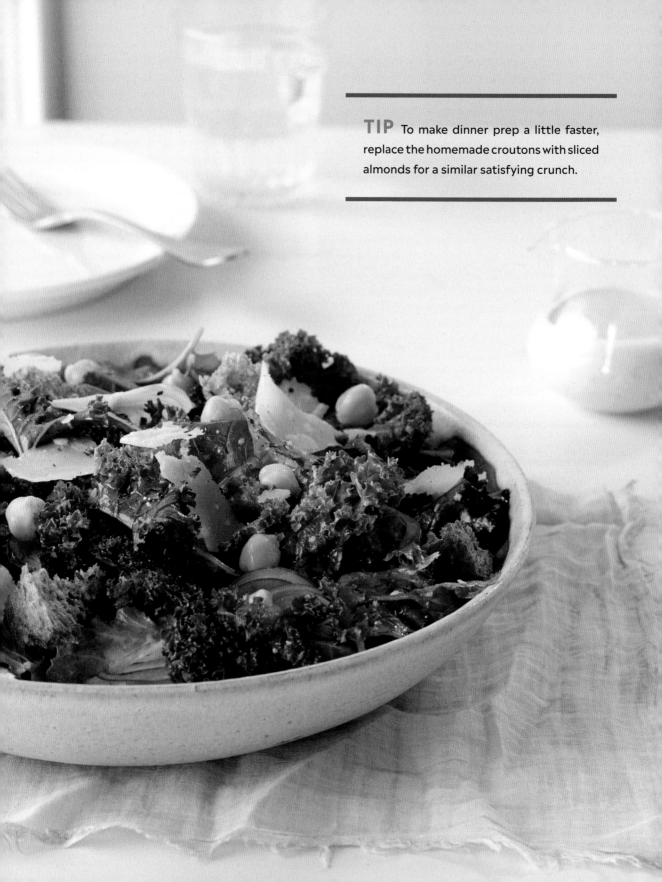

TIP To make dinner prep a little faster, replace the homemade croutons with sliced almonds for a similar satisfying crunch.

KALE CAESAR SALAD

TOTAL TIME: 20 MINUTES ◆ SERVES 4

Kale is one of the most nutrient-dense foods available. A tangy dressing pairs well with its bitter flavor. When purchasing bottled dressing, make sure to review the label to check that there are not added sugars or other undesirable ingredients.

1 large bunch kale, stems removed, leaves torn into bite-size pieces

½ small red onion, thinly sliced

⅓ cup store-bought light Caesar dressing

1 tablespoon olive oil

2 cloves garlic, crushed

2 slices whole-grain bread, torn into bite-size pieces

2 (15-ounce) cans unsalted chickpeas, drained

¼ cup grated or shaved Parmesan cheese

½ teaspoon black pepper

1. Toss kale and onion with dressing until well coated.

2. Heat oil in a medium skillet on medium. Add garlic and cook until fragrant and golden, 2 to 3 minutes.

3. Discard garlic and add bread. Cook, stirring, until bread is golden and crisp, 5 minutes.

4. Add croutons and chickpeas to salad. Sprinkle with cheese and pepper, and toss before serving.

PER SERVING 320 calories, 8 g fat (1.5 g saturated fat), 17 g protein, 440 mg sodium, 48 g carbohydrates, 9 g fiber, 6 g sugars (2 g added sugars), 5 mg cholesterol

SPICED GRILLED EGGPLANT & TOMATO SALAD

TOTAL TIME: 30 MINUTES ◆ SERVES 6

Grilling eggplant brings out the vegetable's natural sugars, making it less bitter and allowing it to stay firm. Eggplant is rich in anthocyanins, which are responsible for the bright pigment of its skin and act as an antioxidant that can protect cells from free radicals.

2 medium eggplants (about 1 pound each), cut lengthwise into ½-inch slices

4 tablespoons olive oil, divided

1 teaspoon ground coriander

1 teaspoon cayenne

½ teaspoon kosher salt

2 tablespoons lemon juice

2 tablespoons red wine vinegar

1½ cups cherry or grape tomatoes in different colors, halved

2 small Fresno chiles or other hot chiles, finely chopped

¼ cup packed mint, finely chopped, plus more for serving

¼ cup plain low-fat Greek yogurt

2 tablespoons low-fat milk

1. Heat grill on medium. Brush eggplant with 3 tablespoons oil, then season with coriander, cayenne, and ¼ teaspoon salt to taste. Grill until tender, 10 to 12 minutes.

2. Meanwhile, in a medium bowl, whisk together lemon juice, vinegar, remaining 1 tablespoon oil, and ¼ teaspoon salt; fold in tomatoes, chiles, and mint.

3. On a large platter, arrange eggplant. Top with tomato salad. In a small bowl, whisk together yogurt and milk; drizzle over vegetables. Sprinkle with more mint, if desired.

PER SERVING 140 calories, 10 g fat (1.5 g saturated fat), 3 g protein, 310 mg sodium, 12 g carbohydrates, 5 g fiber, 6 g sugars (0 g added sugars), 1 mg cholesterol

TIP When you eat foods with lycopene, such as tomatoes, they can stimulate collagen formation to improve your skin's firmness and give you a healthy, youthful glow.

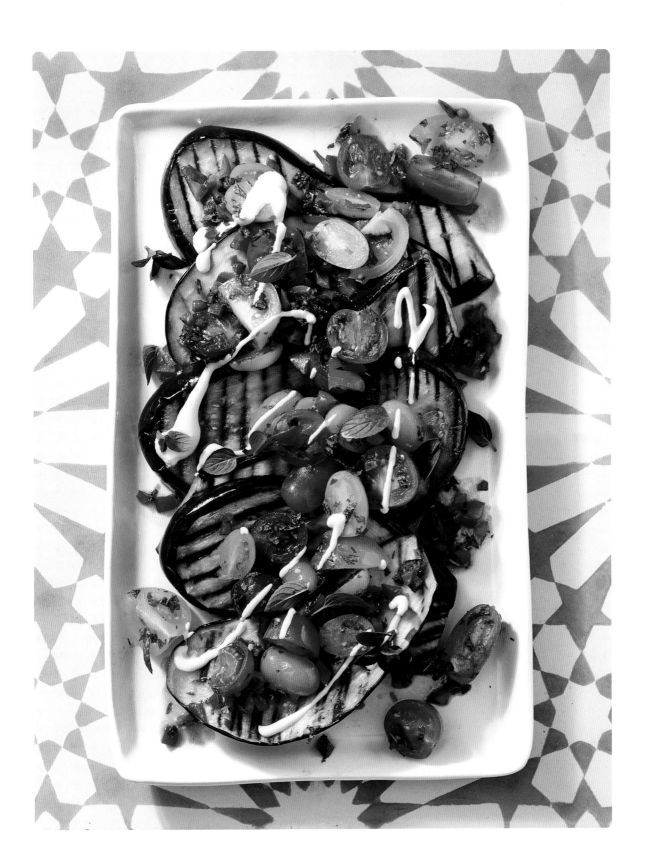

GRILLED VEGGIE & COUSCOUS SALAD

TOTAL TIME: 20 MINUTES ◆ **SERVES 4**

Couscous, a staple in North African cooking, is a tiny pasta made of wheat or barley. But these small pearls pack a nutrient punch, containing more fiber per cup than brown rice and more than half of your daily recommended intake of selenium, a powerful antioxidant that helps fight inflammation and LDL ("bad") cholesterol.

2 medium red peppers, seeded and quartered

2 portobello mushroom caps

2 lemons, halved

5 tablespoons extra virgin olive oil, divided

½ teaspoon plus ¼ teaspoon kosher salt

5 ounces arugula

4 ounces pecorino cheese

1 cup couscous, cooked

¼ teaspoon black pepper

1. Heat grill on medium-high. Brush red peppers, mushroom caps, and lemons with 2 tablespoons oil. Sprinkle with ½ teaspoon salt. Grill mushrooms 15 minutes or until tender, turning once. Grill lemons, cut side down, 8 minutes or until charred. Grill peppers 6 minutes or until softened, turning once.

2. Combine arugula, cheese, couscous, remaining 3 tablespoons oil, remaining ¼ teaspoon salt, and black pepper. Thinly slice peppers and chop mushrooms; add to arugula along with juice from lemons. Toss well.

PER SERVING 450 calories, 23 g fat (7 g saturated fat), 19 g protein, 920 mg sodium, 42 g carbohydrates, 5 g fiber, 5 g sugars (0 g added sugars), 29 mg cholesterol

TIP To keep pesky lemon seeds and charred bits of lemon out of your salad, simply cover the cut side of the lemon with a paper towel before squeezing.

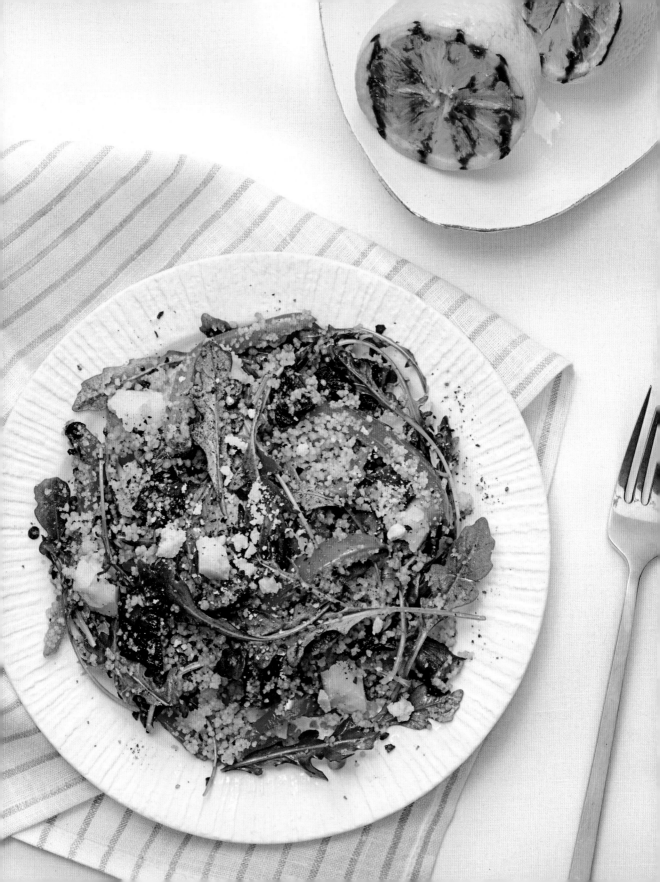

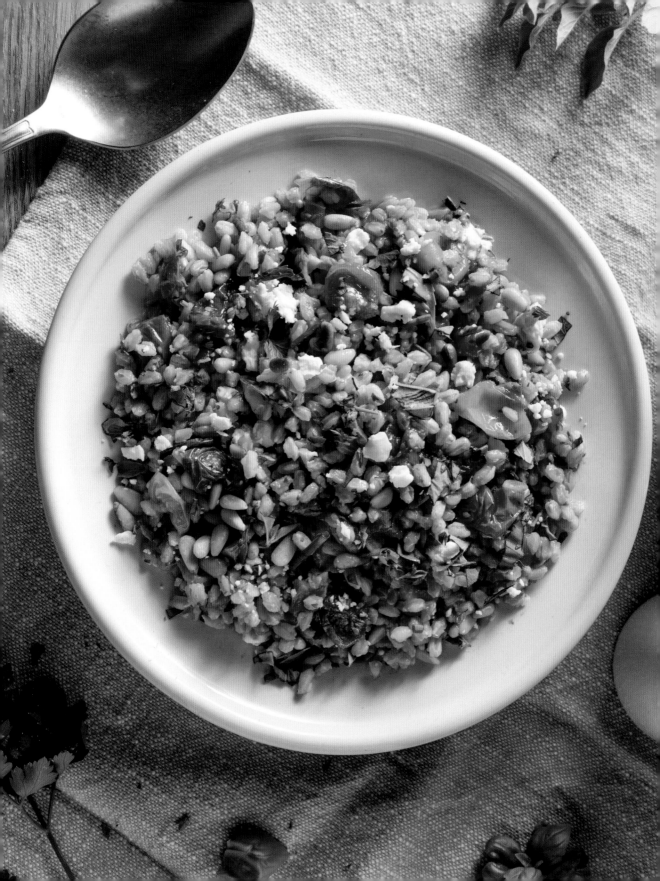

SPELT SALAD WITH APPLES & PINE NUTS

TOTAL TIME: 2 HOURS 15 MINUTES ◆ SERVES 6

With fiber-packed apples tossed with the grains and antimicrobial apple cider vinegar in the dressing, this salad makes the most of the fruit.

1¼ cups spelt or Kamut

1 teaspoon salt

2 large Fuji, Gala, or Braeburn apples, cut into ½-inch chunks

⅓ cup dried currants

¼ cup pine nuts, toasted

2 tablespoons olive oil

2 tablespoons apple cider vinegar

¼ teaspoon black pepper

1. In a large saucepan, combine 4 cups boiling water, spelt, and salt. Bring to a boil again, then reduce to a simmer. Cover and cook until the water has been absorbed, about 1 hour 30 minutes.

2. Transfer cooked spelt to a bowl. Stir in apples, currants, pine nuts, oil, vinegar, and pepper, and toss well. Serve at room temperature or chilled.

PER SERVING 255 calories, 7.5 g fat (1 g saturated fat), 6 g protein, 410 mg sodium, 45 g carbohydrates, 9 g fiber, 16 g sugars, (0 g added sugars), 0 mg cholesterol

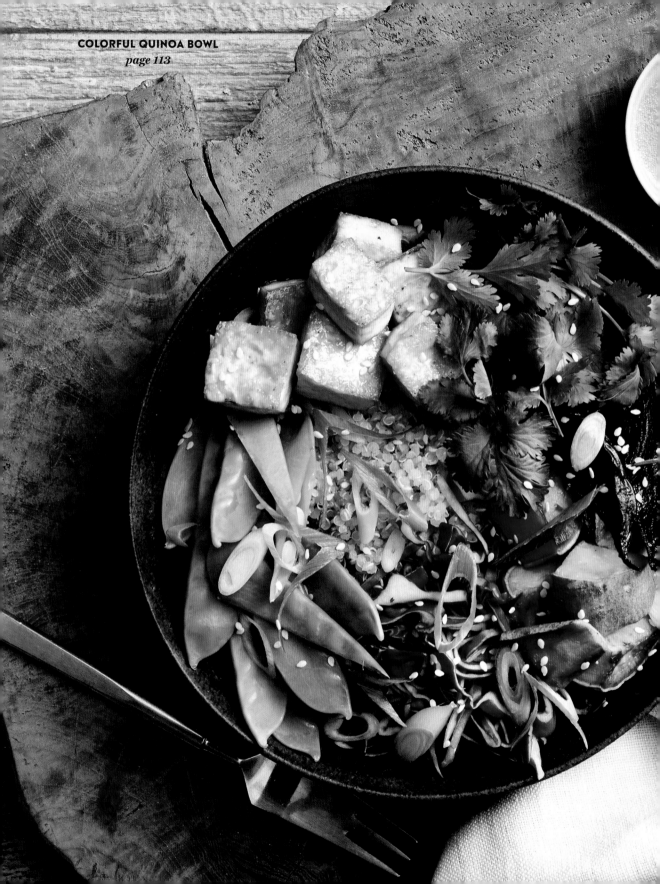

COLORFUL QUINOA BOWL
page 113

Chapter 3

GRAINS & BEANS

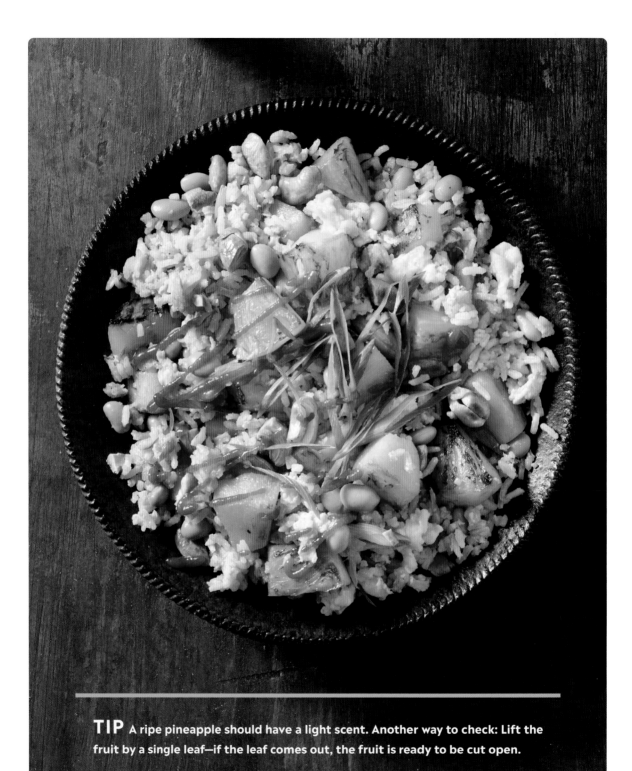

TIP A ripe pineapple should have a light scent. Another way to check: Lift the fruit by a single leaf—if the leaf comes out, the fruit is ready to be cut open.

PINEAPPLE & CASHEW FRIED RICE

TOTAL TIME: 35 MINUTES ◆ SERVES 4

Pineapple is full of bromelain, an enzyme that may help with recovery after exercise and reduce inflammation.

1 tablespoon canola oil

½ small pineapple, peeled, cored, cut into ½-inch chunks (about 2 cups)

1 tablespoon toasted sesame oil

3 cloves garlic, pressed

3 scallions, thinly sliced, white and green parts separated

4 cups cooked long-grain brown rice

2 tablespoons low-sodium soy sauce

1 teaspoon sriracha, plus more for serving

2 large eggs, beaten

½ cup frozen shelled edamame, thawed

½ cup cashews, toasted and chopped

1. Heat canola oil in a large nonstick skillet on medium-high. Add pineapple and cook, tossing occasionally, until golden brown, 3 to 4 minutes; transfer to a plate.

2. Add sesame oil to the skillet along with garlic and scallion whites and cook, tossing, 1 minute. Add rice and cook, tossing occasionally, until heated through, about 3 minutes.

3. Add soy sauce and sriracha, and toss to combine. Push rice to sides of pan, pour eggs into open space, and cook, stirring often, until eggs are almost set, then fold in rice and edamame. Cook until edamame are heated through, about 2 minutes.

4. Toss with cashews and scallion greens; serve with additional sriracha, if desired.

PER SERVING 515 calories, 20 g fat (3.5 g saturated fat), 15 g protein, 360 mg sodium, 72 g carbohydrates, 6 g fiber, 10.5 g sugars (0 g added sugars), 93 mg cholesterol

MISO-EGGPLANT GRAIN BOWL 🌱

TOTAL TIME: 35 MINUTES ◆ SERVES 3

Miso, eggplant, and red cabbage all promote gut health. They offer an abundance of earthy umami flavors in a single protein-rich vegan bowl.

½ cup quinoa, rinsed

¼ cup pearl barley

¼ cup lentils

1 tablespoon white miso

2 teaspoons mirin

1 teaspoon soy sauce

2 tablespoons canola oil, divided

1 small eggplant, diced

2 cups broccoli florets

Salt

2 tablespoons store-bought sesame dressing

½ cup pickled red cabbage, for topping (optional)

1. In a medium pot, combine quinoa, barley, lentils, and 1¾ cup water. Bring to a boil, uncovered, then reduce heat to low. Cover the pot and simmer until grains are tender, 15 to 20 minutes.

2. In a small bowl, whisk together miso, mirin, soy sauce, and 1 teaspoon water.

3. Heat 1 tablespoon oil in a large pan on medium. Add eggplant and cook until browned, 6 to 8 minutes. Add sauce and simmer until thickened, 2 minutes. Transfer cooked eggplant to a plate.

4. Wipe out the pan, add remaining 1 tablespoon oil, and return the pan to medium heat. Add broccoli and sauté until slightly charred and tender, about 3 minutes. Season with salt. Transfer to the plate with eggplant.

5. Toss grains with dressing and divide among 3 bowls. Top each with eggplant and broccoli, plus red cabbage, if desired.

PER SERVING 475 calories, 22 g fat (2 g saturated fat), 18 g protein, 280 mg sodium, 55 g carbohydrates, 16 g fiber, 6 g sugars (1 g added sugars), 0 mg cholesterol

COLORFUL QUINOA BOWL 🌱

This meal has nearly as much filling lean protein as a 3-ounce serving of chicken.

6 tablespoons rice vinegar

¼ cup white miso

¼ cup safflower oil

2 teaspoons peeled and grated ginger

Cooking spray

1 (14-ounce) block firm tofu, pressed dry and cut into 1-inch cubes

1 large sweet potato, cut into 1-inch cubes

2 medium beets, cut into ½-inch wedges

Kosher salt

Black pepper

4 cups cooked quinoa

1½ cups shredded red cabbage

1 cup halved snow peas

1 cup cilantro

2 scallions, sliced

1 tablespoon sesame seeds

1. Heat oven to 425°F. In a bowl, whisk together vinegar, miso, oil, and ginger.

2. Coat 2 baking sheets with cooking spray. Toss tofu in ¼ cup dressing; place on a baking sheet. Season sweet potato and beets with salt and pepper; arrange on the other baking sheet. Roast until tofu is crisp and vegetables are tender, 25 minutes.

3. Divide quinoa among 4 bowls. Top each with tofu, sweet potatoes, beets, cabbage, snow peas, cilantro, scallions, sesame seeds, and remaining dressing.

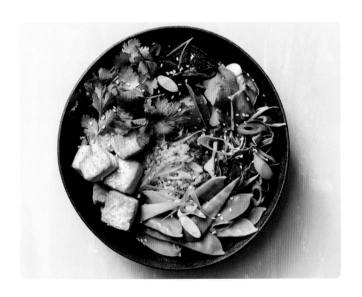

PER SERVING 545 calories, 23 g fat (2 g saturated fat), 21 g protein, 610 mg sodium, 66 g carbohydrates, 12 g fiber, 17 g sugars (0 g added sugars), 0 mg cholesterol

RIGATONI WITH PISTACHIO PESTO

TOTAL TIME: 25 MINUTES ◆ SERVES 6

Combine healthy fats from olive oil with fiber from whole-grain pasta and you get a clean eater's dream. This recipe makes pasta feel fresh again, putting plants at the forefront of the meal.

¾ pound whole-wheat rigatoni

1 cup grated Pecorino Romano cheese, plus more for serving

½ cup shelled pistachios, plus more for serving, chopped

½ cup mint

¼ cup parsley

¼ cup chopped chives, plus more for serving

⅓ cup extra virgin olive oil

1. Cook pasta per package directions; reserve 1 cup pasta water before draining.

2. In a food processor, pulse cheese, pistachios, mint, parsley, and chives while drizzling in oil and ½ cup pasta water in a steady stream. If necessary, add remaining pasta water, 1 tablespoon at a time, until fluid but not runny.

3. Transfer pesto and pasta to a bowl, and toss to coat. Serve with additional cheese, pistachios, and chives.

PER SERVING 465 calories, 24 g fat (6 g saturated fat), 15 g protein, 415 mg sodium, 46 g carbohydrates, 6 g fiber, 3 g sugars (0 g added sugars), 27 mg cholesterol

TIP Pistachios are a good source of fiber, protein, magnesium, copper, vitamin E, folate, and natural cholesterol-lowering compounds called plant sterols. They are also lower in calories than other nuts and packed with antioxidants. Plus, they contain melatonin, which helps regulate the sleep-wake cycle and support brain health.

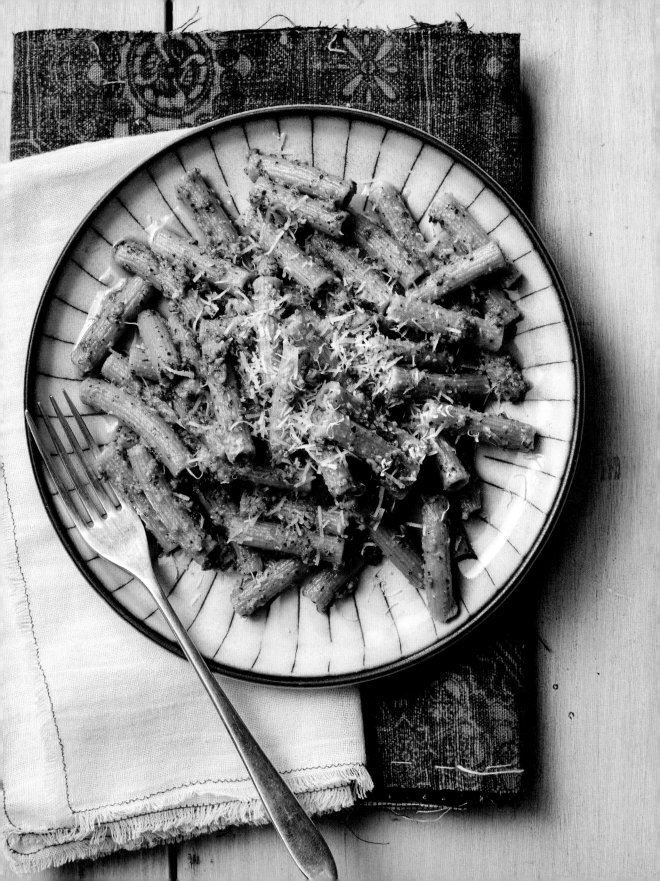

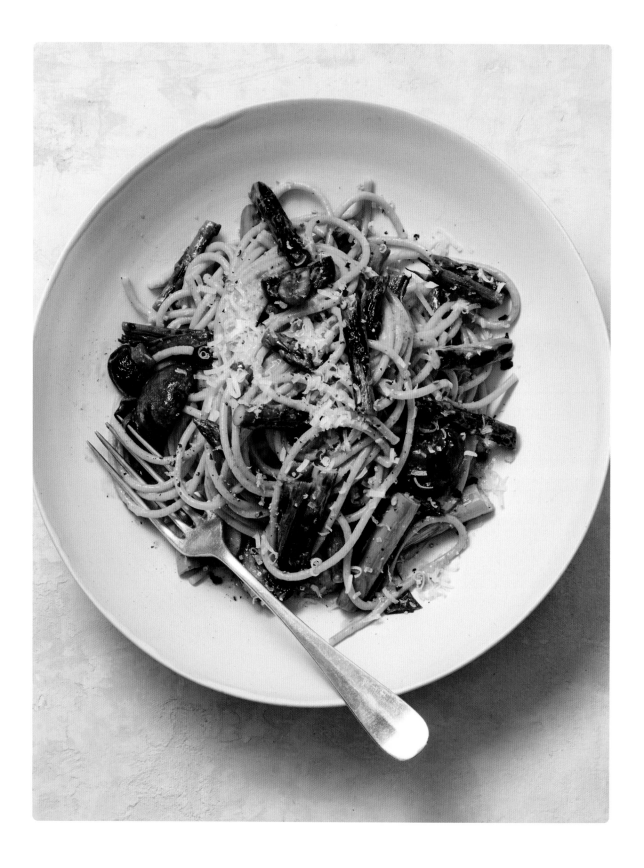

WHOLE-WHEAT SPAGHETTI WITH GRILLED ASPARAGUS & SCALLIONS

TOTAL TIME: 15 MINUTES ◆ **SERVES 4**

That smoky char from the barbecue might taste great, but too much means carcinogenic compounds could be in play. To reduce charring, sear thicker veggies quickly and then lower the temperature to finish cooking.

12 ounces whole-wheat spaghetti

10 ounces mushrooms, sliced

8 ounces asparagus, trimmed

1 bunch scallions, trimmed

1½ tablespoons olive oil

½ teaspoon red pepper flakes

½ teaspoon salt

1 large clove garlic, pressed

2 lemons, zested and halved

Parmesan cheese, grated (optional)

1. Heat grill on medium-high. Cook spaghetti per package directions.

2. In a large bowl, toss mushrooms, asparagus, and scallions with oil, red pepper flakes, and salt. Grill vegetables until just tender, 3 to 5 minutes. Cut asparagus and scallions into 2-inch pieces; return to the bowl.

3. Add garlic and lemon zest to the bowl. Grill lemons, cut side down, until charred.

4. Add spaghetti to the bowl with vegetables, squeeze in juice of grilled lemons, and toss to combine. Serve with cheese, if desired.

PER SERVING 435 calories, 9.5 g fat (1.5 g saturated fat), 18 g protein, 260 mg sodium, 79 g carbohydrates, 12 g fiber, 5.5 g sugars (0 g added sugars), 0 mg cholesterol

SESAME SOBA NOODLES 🌱

TOTAL TIME: 15 MINUTES ◆ SERVES 2

Ginger has been used for its anti-inflammatory, stomach-settling, and pain-relieving properties for thousands of years. Honor that legacy—and treat your ailments as well as your taste buds!—with these earthy noodles.

¼ cup chopped scallions

½ cup sliced portobello mushrooms

3 cups Swiss chard

1 teaspoon peeled and minced ginger

2 teaspoons low-sodium soy sauce

2 teaspoons toasted sesame oil

¼ teaspoon red pepper flakes

2 cups buckwheat noodles

1. In a large nonstick skillet, sauté scallions, mushrooms, Swiss chard, ginger, soy sauce, sesame oil, and red pepper flakes, stirring constantly, 2 to 3 minutes.

2. Meanwhile, cook noodles per package directions; drain.

3. Toss veggies with noodles.

PER SERVING 255 calories, 6 g fat (1 g saturated fat), 8 g protein, 350 mg sodium, 47 g carbohydrates, 4 g fiber, 3 g sugars (0 g added sugars), 0 mg cholesterol

TIP Want a protein boost? Serve this meal with 4 ounces of grilled shrimp, adding 2 ounces to each plate.

SPICY CHICKPEA CROQUETTES ✿

TOTAL TIME: 25 MINUTES ◆ SERVES 4

As if the delicious taste and great texture are not motivators enough, one can of chickpeas contains 25 grams of protein plus 88 percent of your daily fiber and 46 percent of your daily iron.

¾ cup chopped onion

1 clove garlic, chopped

½ red pepper, chopped

1 (15-ounce) can chickpeas

½ teaspoon ground cumin

⅛ teaspoon cayenne

2 tablespoons mint

2 tablespoons lemon juice, divided

¾ teaspoon salt, divided

¾ teaspoon black pepper, divided

All-purpose flour, if needed

5 tablespoons olive oil, divided

8 cups baby spinach

¼ cup minced sun-dried tomatoes

2 tablespoons tahini

1. In a medium skillet on medium-high, sauté onion, garlic, and red pepper until soft, 8 minutes.

2. In a food processor, blend the sautéed vegetables with chickpeas, cumin, cayenne, mint, 1 tablespoon lemon juice, and ¼ teaspoon each salt and black pepper. Form mixture into 8 small patties (add a little flour to bind, if needed).

3. Using the same skillet, heat 2 tablespoons oil on medium-high, and pan-fry patties until golden brown, 6 to 8 minutes per side. Heat 1 tablespoon oil in a separate pan on medium-high, and sauté baby spinach and sun-dried tomatoes; season with ¼ teaspoon each salt and black pepper.

4. Make the sauce: Blend tahini, remaining 2 tablespoons oil, remaining 1 tablespoon lemon juice, 1 tablespoon hot water, and remaining ¼ teaspoon each salt and black pepper. Serve croquettes with sautéed spinach and tahini-lemon sauce.

PER SERVING 350 calories, 23 g fat (3 g saturated fat), 9 g protein, 570 mg sodium, 31 g carbohydrates, 4 g fiber, 6 g sugars (0 g added sugars), 0 mg cholesterol

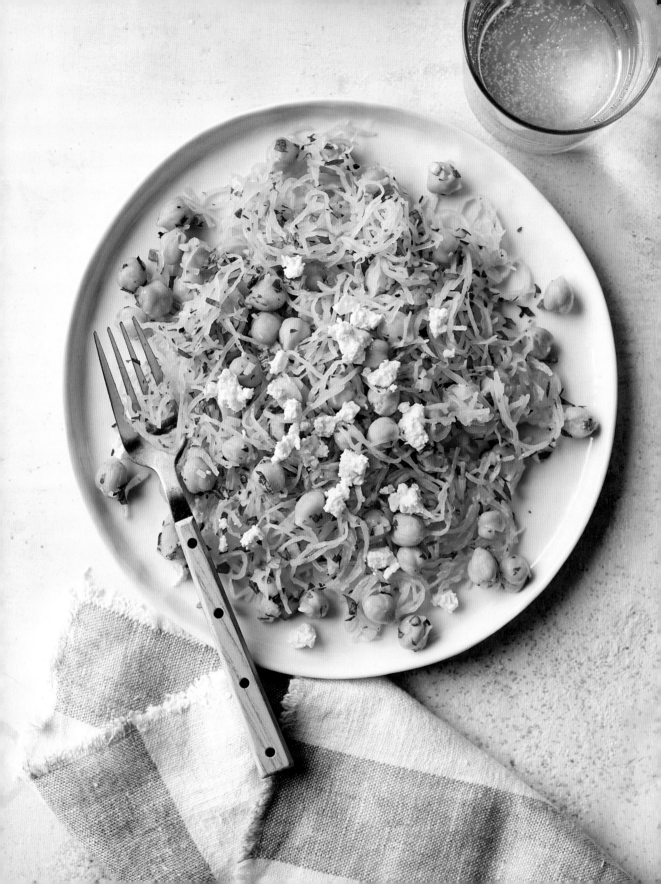

SQUASH & CHICKPEA SAUTÉ

TOTAL TIME: 20 MINUTES ◆ SERVES 4

Spaghetti squash has tons of fiber (one cup has about the same amount of fiber as a small slice of whole-wheat bread), which promotes gut health and better digestion. In this recipe, the squash joins up with protein-rich chickpeas to create a dinner that's guaranteed to leave you satisfied.

1 (3-pound) spaghetti squash

1 small red onion, finely chopped

4 tablespoons lemon juice

Pinch plus ¼ teaspoon kosher salt

Pinch plus ¼ teaspoon black pepper

2 tablespoons olive oil, divided

2 cloves garlic, chopped

1 (15-ounce) can chickpeas, drained and rinsed

1 cup flat-leaf parsley, chopped

2 ounces crumbled feta cheese, for topping

1. Using a large serrated knife, halve spaghetti squash lengthwise; discard seeds. Place halves cut side down on a large piece of parchment paper and microwave on high power until just tender, 9 to 11 minutes. Use a fork to shred squash strands; transfer to a large bowl.

2. In a small bowl, toss onion, lemon juice, and a pinch each salt and pepper.

3. Heat 1 tablespoon oil in a nonstick skillet. Add garlic and cook until beginning to turn golden brown. Add chickpeas and cook, 2 minutes. Toss with spaghetti squash, remaining 1 tablespoon oil, and ¼ teaspoon each salt and pepper. Fold in parsley plus onion mixture (including juices). Top with cheese.

PER SERVING 245 calories, 10 g fat (1.5 g fat), 7 g protein, 340 mg sodium, 27 g carbohydrates, 8 g fiber, 11 g sugars (0 g added sugars), 13 mg cholesterol

TWO-BEAN HARVEST CHILI

TOTAL TIME: 35 MINUTES ◆ SERVES 4

Beans have the highest antioxidant count of any food, and they fill you up fast. Black beans provide a valuable source of resistant starch, which helps keep blood glucose levels on an even keel.

2 teaspoons vegetable oil

1 large (10- to 12-ounce) onion, finely chopped

12 ounces carrots, finely chopped (about 2 cups)

4 cloves garlic, chopped

½ teaspoon salt, divided

1 (6-ounce) bunch collard greens, stems and tough ribs discarded, leaves chopped

1 tablespoon salt-free chili powder

1 teaspoon ground cumin

¼ teaspoon dried oregano

1 (28-ounce) can no-salt-added diced tomatoes

2 (15-ounce) cans no-salt-added beans, preferably black beans and pink beans, drained and rinsed

¼ cup reduced-fat sour cream, for topping

1. Heat oil in a 6-quart saucepot on medium. Add onion, carrots, garlic, and ¼ teaspoon salt. Cook 8 to 10 minutes or until golden and tender, stirring occasionally.

2. Add collard greens and remaining ¼ teaspoon salt and cook 1 to 2 minutes, stirring, until collards are bright green and just tender. Stir in chili powder, cumin, and oregano and cook 1 minute, stirring.

3. Stir in tomatoes and beans. Simmer 10 minutes, stirring occasionally. Divide among 4 bowls; top with sour cream.

PER SERVING 335 calories, 5 g fat (2 g saturated fat), 16 g protein, 410 mg sodium, 58 g carbohydrates, 17 g fiber, 13 g sugars (0 g added sugars), 8 mg cholesterol

TIP One cup of beans provides a whopping 13 grams of fiber and 15 grams of protein.

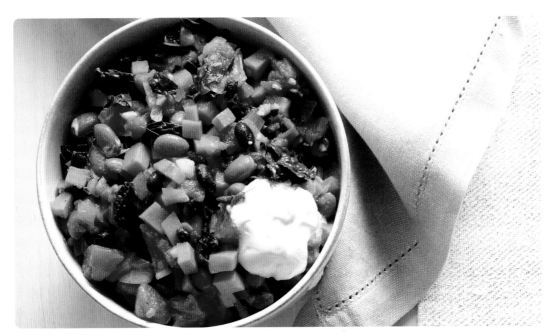

BEANS 101: SHOPPING TIPS

Beans are a plant-based protein powerhouse and a staple of this eating plan (added bonus: bean eaters have an amazing 22 percent lower risk of obesity). Keep these tips in mind when shopping for these mighty plants.

Buy canned: They're just as healthy.

You may have heard that dried beans are best, but they need to be soaked overnight, then boiled for hours before they're ready to eat. Who has the time or patience for that? Bagged beans are generally less expensive and have no added ingredients, including salt. But canned varieties, which are ready to eat, can be just as nutritious.

Go for low sodium.

Low-sodium canned beans are exactly the same price as salted canned beans, with two-thirds less sodium. That's a decrease from about 720 milligrams per cup (a third of the daily max of 2,300 mg) to 220 milligrams. Rinsing beans in a colander under cold water for one minute will wash away about a quarter of the sodium too.

Look for vegetarian versions.

Baked and refried varieties are traditionally prepared with lard or bits of pork, which add calories, cholesterol, sodium, and saturated fat. Choosing vegetarian refried beans reduces the saturated fat content from 16 percent of the daily value to zero per cup, and adds a bonus 2 grams of protein—and they taste just as delicious.

Avoid dented or bulging cans.

Small dents and dings are OK, but if you find a badly dented or swollen can in your cupboard, or if a can spurts liquid when opened, toss it out right away. These are all possible signs of botulism, a potentially deadly form of food poisoning. If you're ever unsure, think, *When in doubt, throw it out.*

FARRO WITH WILD MUSHROOM DRESSING ✿

TOTAL TIME: 1 HOUR ◆ SERVES 8

Subbing mushrooms for traditional sausage gives this hearty, fiber-full dish all the flavor you love but with a fraction of the sodium and saturated fat.

2 tablespoons red quinoa

¼ teaspoon plus 4 tablespoons olive oil, divided

1 medium onion, chopped

1 medium leek, white and light-green parts only, cut into ¼-inch half-moons

¾ teaspoon kosher salt, divided

¾ teaspoon black pepper, divided

2½ cups farro

5 cups low-sodium vegetable or chicken broth

2 sprigs rosemary

1½ pounds wild mushrooms, trimmed and sliced

4 cloves garlic, finely chopped

1 bunch spinach, thick stems discarded (about 4 cups)

1. Heat oven to 350°F. On a small baking sheet, toss quinoa with ¼ teaspoon oil and bake until toasted and nutty-smelling, 5 to 7 minutes; set aside.

2. Heat 1 tablespoon oil in a Dutch oven on medium. Add onion and cook, covered, stirring occasionally, 5 minutes. Add leek, season with ½ teaspoon each salt and pepper, and cook, stirring occasionally, until vegetables begin to soften, 5 to 6 minutes.

3. Transfer half the onion mixture to a small bowl. Add farro to the Dutch oven and cook, stirring, 1 minute. Add broth and rosemary and bring to a boil. Reduce heat and simmer, covered, until liquid has been absorbed, 30 to 35 minutes. Remove from heat and let sit, covered, 5 minutes. Discard rosemary and fluff.

4. Heat 2 tablespoons oil in a large skillet on medium-high. Add half the mushrooms, season with ¼ teaspoon each salt and pepper, and cook, tossing occasionally, until golden brown and tender, 5 to 6 minutes. Add 2 cloves garlic and cook, tossing, 1 minute; transfer to a large bowl. Repeat with remaining 1 tablespoon oil, mushrooms, and garlic. Add farro, spinach, and reserved onions to the large bowl, and toss to combine.

PER SERVING 350 calories, 9.5 g fat (1.5 g saturated fat), 15 g protein, 250 mg sodium, 55 g carbohydrates, 9 g fiber, 3 g sugars (0 g added sugars), 0 mg cholesterol

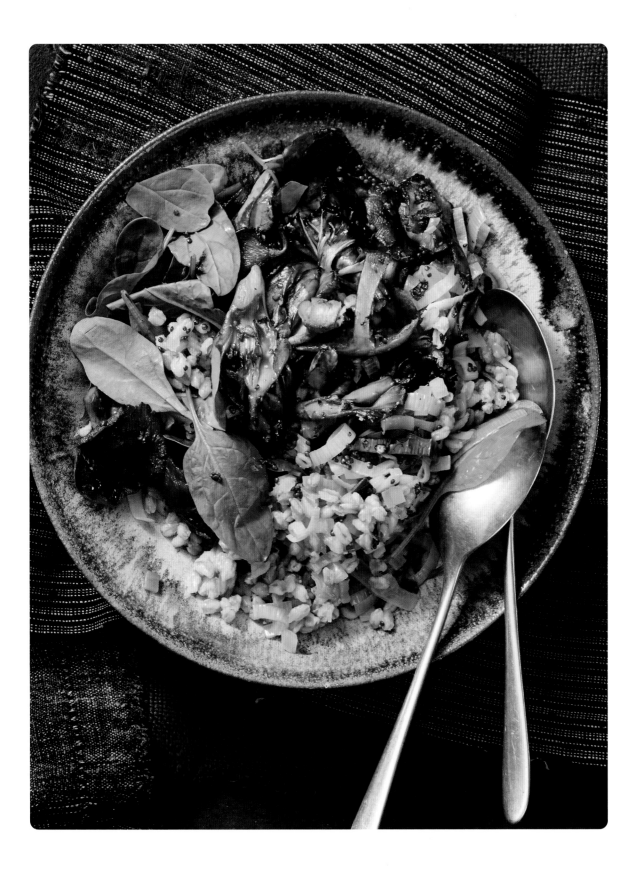

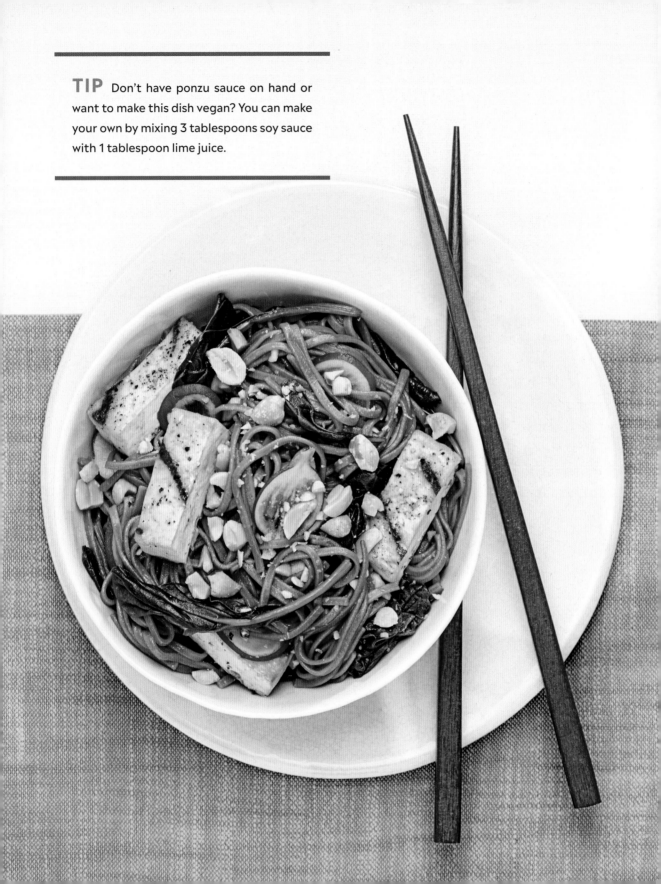

TIP Don't have ponzu sauce on hand or want to make this dish vegan? You can make your own by mixing 3 tablespoons soy sauce with 1 tablespoon lime juice.

SOBA NOODLES WITH GRILLED TOFU

TOTAL TIME: 25 MINUTES ◆ SERVES 4

Japanese ponzu sauce, with a tart, tangy flavor that's akin to a vinaigrette, takes this vegan dish to another level. And don't skip the radishes—besides adding crunch, they're chock-full of vitamins A, B6, C, E, and K.

12 ounces extra-firm tofu

¼ teaspoon kosher salt

¼ teaspoon black pepper

8 ounces soba noodles

5 ounces baby spinach

¼ cup ponzu sauce

6 radishes, thinly sliced

¼ cup peanuts, chopped, for topping

1. Heat grill or grill pan on medium-high. Cut tofu into ½-inch slices; press dry with paper towels. Season with salt and pepper.

2. Grill tofu, covered, 10 to 15 minutes, turning once. Cut into bite-size pieces.

3. Meanwhile, cook noodles per package directions. Place baby spinach in colander in sink; drain cooked noodles directly over spinach. Rinse noodles and spinach with cold water; drain well.

4. In a large bowl, toss noodles and spinach with ponzu sauce, radishes, and grilled tofu. Top with peanuts.

PER SERVING 360 calories, 10 g fat (1 g saturated fat), 18 g protein, 775 mg sodium, 51 g carbohydrates, 6 g fiber, 3 g sugars (2 g added sugars), 0 mg cholesterol

GRAPEFRUIT COUSCOUS WITH CANNELLINI BEANS

TOTAL TIME: 15 MINUTES ◆ SERVES 4

Mild couscous, tangy feta, and tart grapefruit make a perfect trio of contrasts in this light, summery salad. Beyond the vitamin C that citrus is famous for, grapefruit is a great source of nutrients that have been shown to aid in weight loss, prevent diabetes, and promote appetite control.

1 (7.6-ounce) box couscous

2 tablespoons olive oil

1 tablespoon red wine vinegar

¼ teaspoon salt

¼ teaspoon black pepper

½ (15-ounce) can cannellini beans, drained and rinsed (about 1 cup)

2 ounces crumbled feta cheese

1 grapefruit, peeled and sectioned

¼ cup mint, for topping

1. Cook couscous per package directions. Transfer to a large bowl.

2. Toss couscous with oil, vinegar, salt, and pepper. Stir in beans, cheese, and grapefruit. Top with mint.

PER SERVING 490 calories, 11 g fat (3 g saturated fat), 16 g protein, 355 mg sodium, 82 g carbohydrates, 7 g fiber, 7 g sugars (0 g added sugars), 13 mg cholesterol

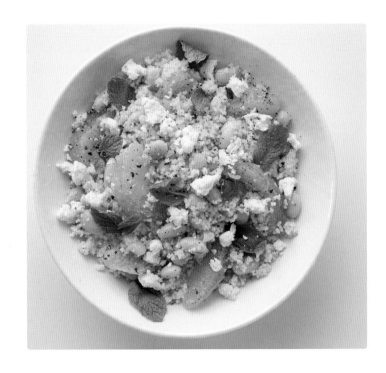

LEMON ORZO WITH ZUCCHINI

TOTAL TIME: 25 MINUTES ◆ **SERVES 4**

When you can't choose between rice and pasta, orzo is always there to split the difference. For this dish, make sure you use a whole-wheat variety, as it pairs well with the mild, antioxidant-rich zucchini.

8 ounces whole-wheat orzo

12 ounces zucchini, shredded (about 3 cups)

1 tablespoon lemon zest

3 tablespoons lemon juice

1 tablespoon olive oil

¼ teaspoon kosher salt

¼ teaspoon black pepper

3 tablespoons grated Parmesan cheese

½ cup basil, chopped

¼ cup roughly chopped chives

1. Cook orzo per package directions. Drain into a colander and immediately fold in zucchini. Let sit 1 minute.

2. Transfer zucchini-orzo mixture to a bowl and toss with lemon zest and juice, oil, salt, and pepper; let cool completely.

3. Toss with cheese, then fold in basil and chives before serving.

PER SERVING 260 calories, 6 g fat (1 g saturated fat), 11 g protein, 200 mg sodium, 46 g carbohydrates, 5 g fiber, 4 g sugars (0 g added sugars), 3 mg cholesterol

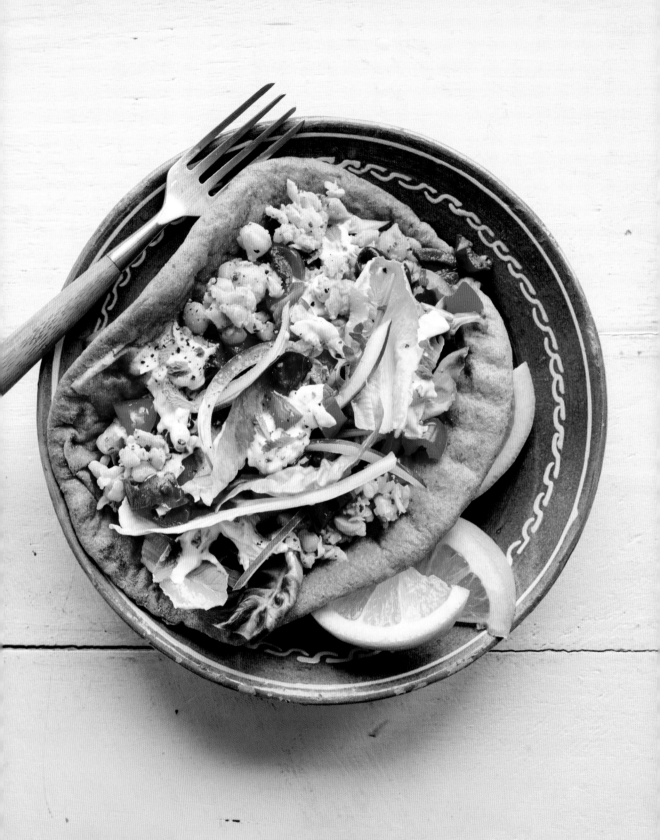

BLACK BEAN & CORN TOSTADAS

TOTAL TIME: 15 MINUTES ◆ SERVES 4

Want to whip up your own salsa for this dish? Make the jalapeño-poblano salsa verde on page 194. The cranberry salsa on page 187 would also work and be a bit unexpected!

4 (6-inch) corn tortillas

1 (15-ounce) can black beans, drained and rinsed

¼ cup salsa

½ cup canned corn kernels, drained

1 avocado, diced

½ cup crumbled feta cheese

½ cup shredded red cabbage

Lime wedges, for serving

1. Heat oven to 375°F. On a baking sheet, arrange corn tortillas. Bake until crisp, 3 minutes per side.

2. In a pan, heat black beans on medium-high. Add salsa and cook, stirring, until heated through.

3. In a small bowl, mash beans and spread on warmed tortillas. Divide corn, avocado, cheese, and cabbage among tortillas. Finish each tostada with a squeeze of lime juice.

PER SERVING 300 calories, 12 g fat (4 g saturated fat), 11 g protein, 450 mg sodium, 39 g carbohydrates, 10 g fiber, 6 g sugars (1 g added sugars), 17 mg cholesterol

GREEK CHICKPEA TACOS

TOTAL TIME: 20 MINUTES ◆ SERVES 4

Bring the Mediterranean diet to taco night: This healthful twist features probiotic-rich Greek yogurt, stomach-soothing mint, and 10 grams of fiber per serving.

1 (15-ounce) can unsalted chickpeas, drained and rinsed

2 tablespoons lemon juice, divided

2 tablespoons olive oil

1 teaspoon dried oregano

4 (6-inch) whole-wheat pitas, warmed

2 cups mixed spring greens

1 large tomato, diced

½ small red onion, thinly sliced

¼ cup pitted kalamata olives, sliced

½ seedless cucumber, peeled and grated, plus diced cucumber for serving

1 cup plain Greek yogurt

2 tablespoons chopped mint, plus leaves for serving

1 clove garlic, minced

Kosher salt

1. In a medium bowl, mash chickpeas with 1 tablespoon lemon juice, oil, and oregano. Spread a quarter of the mixture on each pita. Top with greens, tomato, onion, and olives.

2. In a medium bowl, combine grated cucumber, yogurt, mint, remaining 1 tablespoon lemon juice, garlic, and a pinch of salt. Drizzle over taco fillings. Top with more mint and diced cucumber, if desired.

PER SERVING 430 calories, 16.5 g fat (3.5 g saturated fat), 17 g protein, 695 mg sodium, 58 g carbohydrates, 10 g fiber, 6 g sugars (0 g added sugars), 8 mg cholesterol

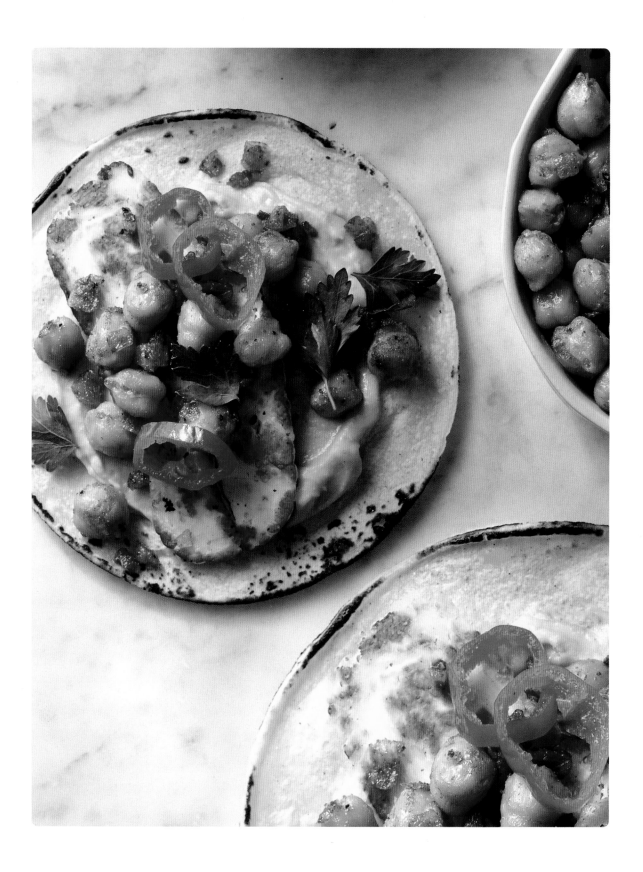

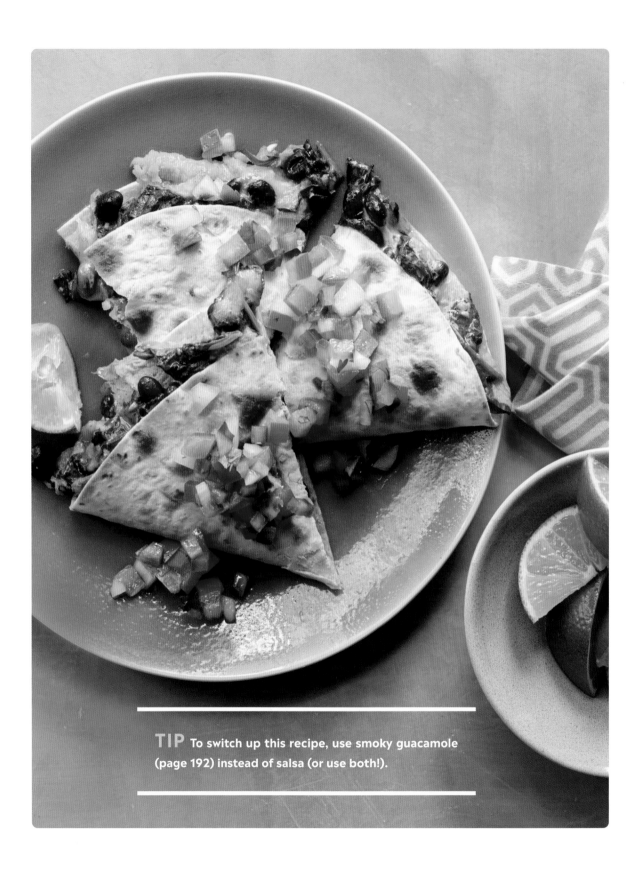

TIP To switch up this recipe, use smoky guacamole (page 192) instead of salsa (or use both!).

SWEET POTATO, BLACK BEAN & SPINACH QUESADILLAS

TOTAL TIME: 20 MINUTES ◆ SERVES 4

We combined these ingredients because they work together, both flavor-wise and nutritionally: The vitamin C in the sweet potatoes helps your body absorb the plant-based iron from the spinach.

12 ounces small sweet potatoes (about 2), halved lengthwise

2 tablespoons olive oil

2 cloves garlic, finely chopped

1 teaspoon ground cumin

½ teaspoon cinnamon

¼ teaspoon cayenne

1 (15-ounce) can low-sodium black beans, drained and rinsed

1 bunch spinach, thick stems discarded, leaves roughly chopped

4 medium tortillas

3 ounces Jack cheese, grated

Lime wedges and salsa, for serving

1. Heat broiler. Line a large broiler-proof baking sheet with foil. Place sweet potatoes on a plate, cut side down, and microwave on high until tender, 5 to 7 minutes.

2. Heat oil in a large skillet on medium. Add garlic and cook until sizzling. Stir in cumin, cinnamon, and cayenne; cook 30 seconds.

3. Add beans and ⅓ cup water and cook, tossing occasionally, until heated through, about 2 minutes. Add spinach and cook, tossing, 1 minute; remove from heat.

4. Place tortillas on the prepared baking sheet. Scoop sweet potato from skins and spread on one half of each tortilla. Top with bean mixture and cheese, then fold over tortillas to cover filling (they will look overstuffed). Broil until tops are golden brown and cheese has melted, about 2 minutes. Serve with lime wedges and salsa, if desired.

PER SERVING 445 calories, 17.5 g fat (6.5 g saturated fat), 18 g protein, 730 mg sodium, 55 g carbohydrates, 11 g fiber, 5 g sugars (0 g added sugars), 49 mg cholesterol

BLACK BEAN CHILI WITH MACARONI

TOTAL TIME: 25 MINUTES ◆ SERVES 6

Following a plant-based regimen starts with small steps. This chili, which is full of plant-based protein and fiber from black beans plus anti-inflammatory chili powder, is a good place for you to begin.

1 medium onion, chopped

2 tablespoons chili powder

1 tablespoon canola oil

½ teaspoon salt

1 (28-ounce) can crushed tomatoes

1 (15-ounce) can black beans, drained and rinsed

1 pound macaroni, cooked

1 cup shredded sharp Cheddar cheese

Chopped cilantro, for topping

1. In a large pot on medium heat, combine onion, chili powder, oil, and salt; cook, stirring often, 8 minute. Add crushed tomatoes and black beans.

2. Heat to simmer, and cook 5 minutes. Toss with macaroni and cheese. Top with cilantro.

PER SERVING 500 calories, 11 g fat (4 g saturated fat), 22 g protein, 770 mg sodium, 82 g carbohydrates, 11 g fiber, 8 g sugars (0 g added sugars), 17 mg cholesterol

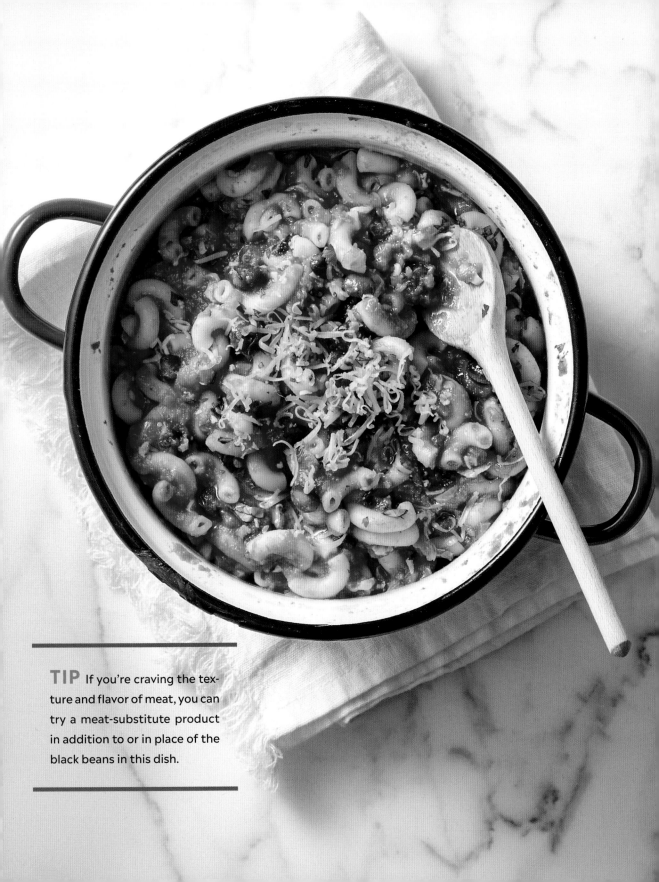

TIP If you're craving the texture and flavor of meat, you can try a meat-substitute product in addition to or in place of the black beans in this dish.

TAHINI-LEMON QUINOA WITH ASPARAGUS RIBBONS ✿

TOTAL TIME: 45 MINUTES   ◆   SERVES 4

Here's a vegan recipe made entirely with whole foods, from vitamin-C-rich lemon to folate-packed asparagus. But the real scene-stealer is the tahini sauce, which offers healthy fats and has been linked to lowering cancer rates.

1 (15-ounce) can chickpeas, drained and rinsed

1 lemon, zested and juiced

Kosher salt

¼ teaspoon black pepper

1 cup quinoa

½ cup tahini

¼ cup lime juice

1 tablespoon honey or agave

1 cup packed mint leaves

1 pound thick asparagus

¼ cup shelled pistachios, chopped, for topping

1. In a bowl, combine chickpeas, lemon zest and juice, salt to taste, and pepper. Let sit 20 minutes or refrigerate overnight, then drain.

2. Meanwhile, cook quinoa per package directions and season with salt to taste.

3. In a blender, puree tahini, lime juice, honey, mint, ½ cup water, and ¼ teaspoon salt until smooth, adding additional water if needed.

4. With vegetable peeler, shave asparagus into ribbons, working from woody end toward tip. In a bowl, combine cooked quinoa, asparagus ribbons, and marinated chickpeas. Sprinkle with pistachios and drizzle with tahini dressing.

PER SERVING 525 calories, 24 g fat (3 g saturated fat), 20 g protein, 315 mg sodium, 64 g carbohydrates, 13 g fiber, 11 g sugars (4 g added sugars), 0 mg cholesterol

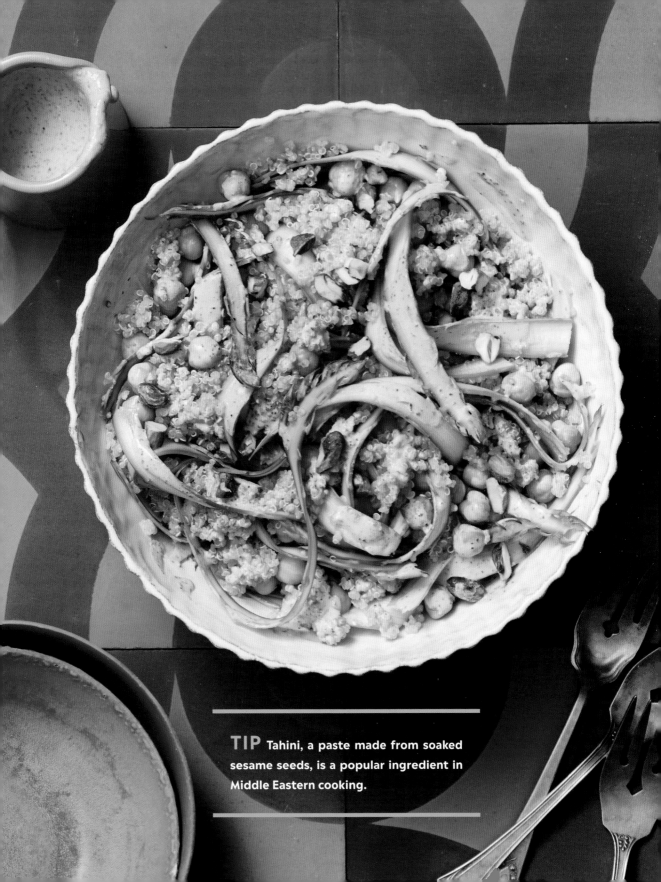

TIP Tahini, a paste made from soaked sesame seeds, is a popular ingredient in Middle Eastern cooking.

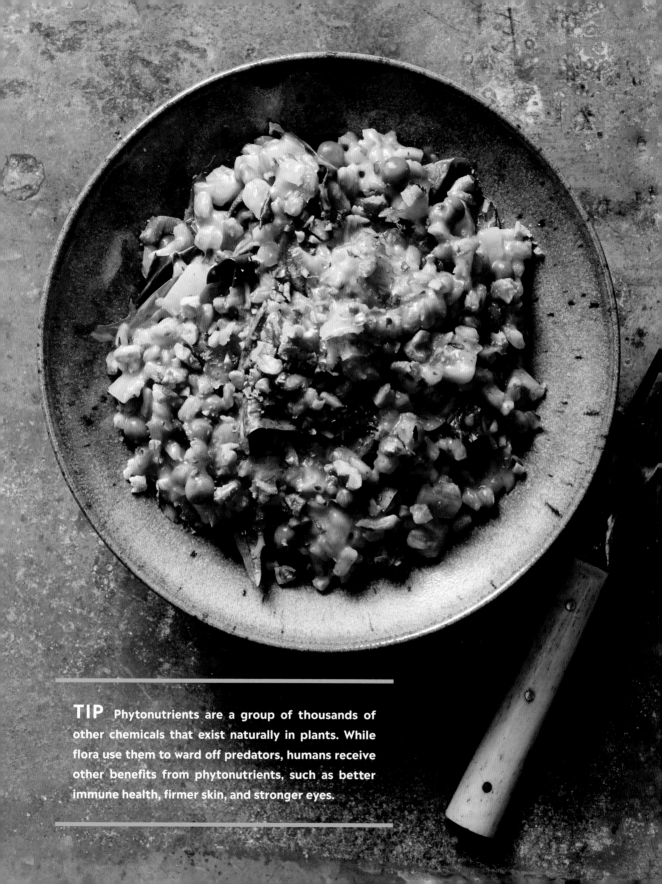

TIP Phytonutrients are a group of thousands of other chemicals that exist naturally in plants. While flora use them to ward off predators, humans receive other benefits from phytonutrients, such as better immune health, firmer skin, and stronger eyes.

FARRO RISOTTO WITH FENNEL, PEAS & GREENS 🌿

Farro is a nutty whole grain that makes a delicious base for this risotto-type dish. Fennel stimulates digestion, while peas and dandelion greens deliver essential vitamins, minerals, and phytonutrients.

1 (13.5-ounce) can light coconut milk

1 cup pearled farro

½ cup reduced-sodium vegetable broth

½ cup dry white wine

½ small yellow onion, diced

1 small fennel bulb, diced

3 tablespoons olive oil

2 tablespoons chopped thyme

1 teaspoon kosher salt

3 cups trimmed and chopped dandelion greens

1 cup frozen peas, thawed

¼ cup finely chopped toasted walnuts, for topping

1. In a 6-quart slow cooker, combine coconut milk, farro, broth, wine, onion, fennel, oil, thyme, and salt. Cover and cook on high until farro and vegetables are tender, 3 to 4 hours.

2. Stir in greens and peas, cover, and continue cooking until greens are wilted, about 20 minutes. Serve topped with walnuts.

PER SERVING 305 calories, 14 g fat (4 g saturated fat), 8 g protein, 465 mg sodium, 38 g carbohydrates, 8 g fiber, 4 g sugars (0 g added sugars), 0 mg cholesterol

GUAVA BARBECUE SAUCE & PULLED JACKFRUIT SANDWICH
page 148

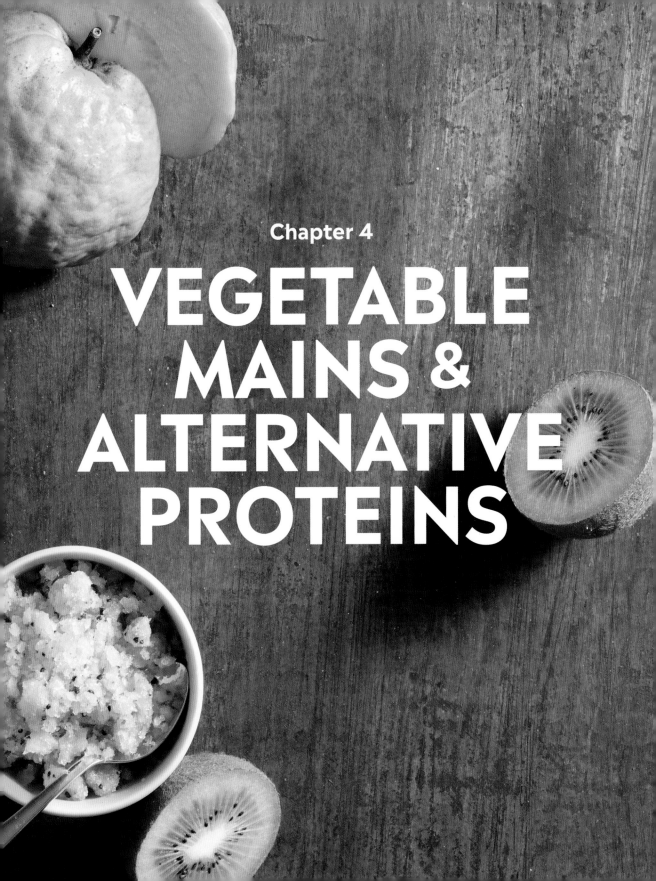

Chapter 4

VEGETABLE MAINS & ALTERNATIVE PROTEINS

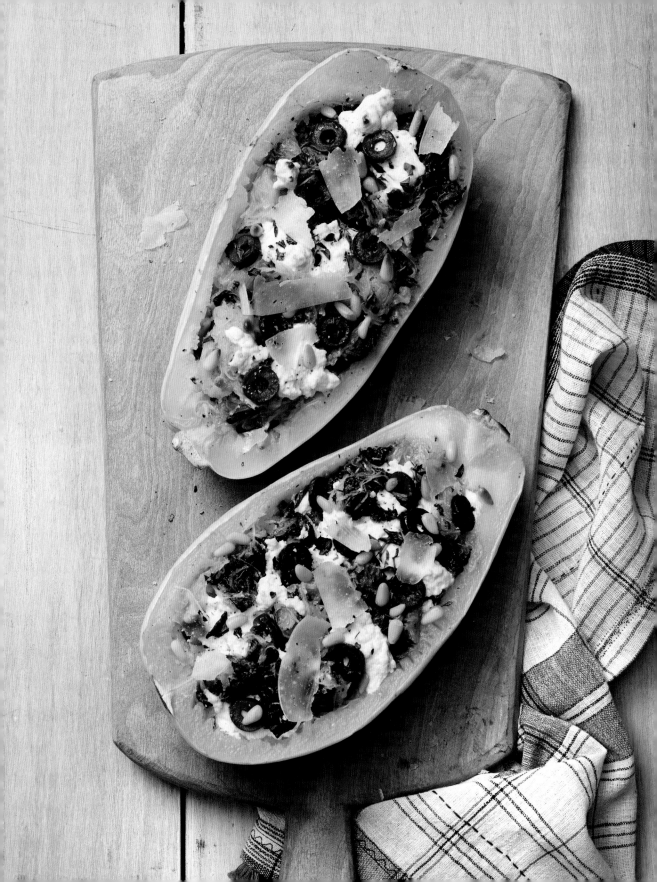

SPAGHETTI SQUASH BOATS

TOTAL TIME: 1 HOUR 20 MINUTES ◆ SERVES 4

A great noodle alternative, spaghetti squash becomes slightly sweet when roasted. It is low in calories, high in fiber, and helpful in keeping your digestion on track. These bowls, assembled and served in the squash shells, are about as whole as whole foods can get.

2 small spaghetti squash (about 3 pounds each), halved and seeded

16 ounces part-skim ricotta

10 ounces frozen chopped spinach, thawed and squeezed dry

¼ cup sliced pitted kalamata olives

2 tablespoons chopped oregano

4 teaspoons lemon zest

4 teaspoons olive oil

½ teaspoon kosher salt

½ teaspoon black pepper

4 teaspoons pine nuts, toasted

1 ounce pecorino, shaved

1. Heat oven to 425°F. Place squash halves, cut side down, on a baking sheet. Add 2 cups water and cover tightly with foil. Bake until squash is tender, 30 minutes.

2. Cool slightly. Using a fork, scrape squash flesh into a bowl. Stir in ricotta, spinach, olives, oregano, lemon zest, oil, salt, and pepper.

3. Divide mixture among 4 squash halves, and bake until bubbly, 20 minutes more. Garnish with pine nuts and pecorino before serving.

PER SERVING 385 calories, 25 g fat (8 g saturated fat), 20 g protein, 915 mg sodium, 24 g carbohydrates, 5 g fiber, 5 g sugars (0 g added sugars), 45 mg cholesterol

TIP You'll know your spaghetti squash is ripe when it has an even, matte yellow color all across its hard husk. If there are any green or glossy spots, give it some more time to mature.

ROASTED CAULIFLOWER "STEAK" SALAD

TOTAL TIME: 1 HOUR ◆ **SERVES 4**

When shopping for dandelion greens, look for the younger, smaller ones found in the spring. If only bunches of the larger variety are available (and you don't like their extra-bitter bite), opt for arugula instead.

2 tablespoons olive oil, divided

2 large heads cauliflower (about 3 pounds each), trimmed of outer leaves

2 teaspoons za'atar

1½ teaspoons kosher salt, divided

1¼ teaspoons black pepper, divided

1 teaspoon ground cumin

2 large carrots

8 ounces dandelion greens, tough stems removed

½ cup plain low-fat Greek yogurt

2 tablespoons tahini

2 tablespoons lemon juice

1 garlic clove, minced

1. Heat oven to 450°F. Brush a large baking sheet with about ½ tablespoon oil.

2. Place cauliflower on cutting board, stem side down. Cut down middle, through core and stem, and then cut two 1-inch "steaks" from middle. Repeat with other cauliflower head. Reserve remaining cauliflower for another use. Brush both sides of steaks with remaining 1½ tablespoons oil, and set on the baking sheet.

3. Combine za'atar, 1 teaspoon each salt and pepper, and cumin. Sprinkle on cauliflower steaks. Bake until bottom is deep golden brown, about 30 minutes. Flip and bake until tender, 10 to 15 minutes.

4. Meanwhile, set carrots on cutting board and use vegetable peeler to peel into ribbons. Add to a large bowl with dandelion greens.

5. In a small bowl, combine yogurt, tahini, lemon juice, 1 tablespoon water, garlic, remaining ½ teaspoon salt, and remaining ¼ teaspoon pepper.

6. Dab 3 tablespoons of the dressing onto the carrot-dandelion mix. With spoon or your hands, massage dressing into mix, 5 minutes.

7. Remove steaks from oven and transfer to individual plates. Drizzle each with 2 tablespoons dressing and top with 1 cup salad.

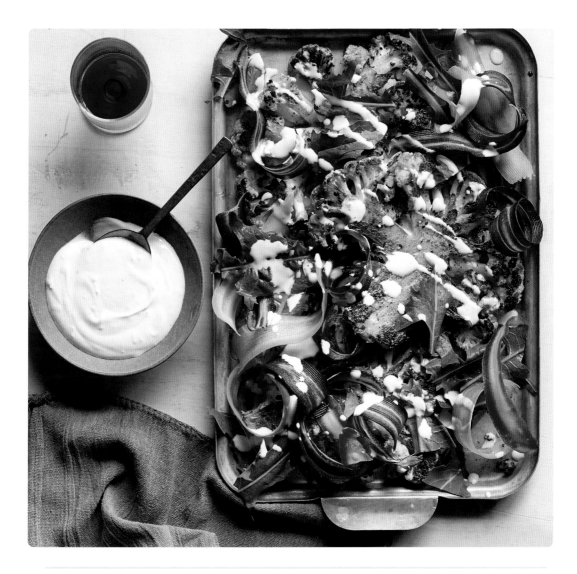

PER SERVING 215 calories, 12 g fat (2 g saturated fat), 9 g protein, 850 mg sodium, 21 g carbohydrates, 7 g fiber, 8 g sugars (0 g added sugars), 2 mg cholesterol

TIP Cruciferous vegetables such as cauliflower, broccoli, cabbage, and Brussels sprouts are filled with antioxidants, including vitamin C and plant compounds called carotenoids, which are particularly powerful brain protectors. A Harvard Medical School study of more than 13,000 women found that those who ate the more cruciferous vegetables lowered their brain age by one to two years.

GUAVA BARBECUE SAUCE & PULLED JACKFRUIT SANDWICH

TOTAL TIME: 55 MINUTES ◆ SERVES 4

This sandwich is a tasty and super-healthy alternative to pulled pork. Jackfruit's mild flavor makes it a good substitute for meat, while guava is chock-full of vitamin C, protein, and fiber.

1 tablespoon olive oil

1 small yellow onion, thinly sliced

2 cloves garlic, sliced

2 teaspoons peeled and grated ginger

½ cup guava paste

1 tablespoon apple cider vinegar

2 tablespoons spiced rum

1 tablespoon tomato paste

2 teaspoons low-sodium soy sauce

1 teaspoon Worcestershire sauce

¾ teaspoon kosher salt, divided

1 (20-ounce) can young green jackfruit in water (not syrup), drained and rinsed

1 jalapeño, thinly sliced

¼ red onion, thinly sliced

2 tablespoons lime juice

4 whole-wheat buns

1 ripe avocado, thinly sliced, for topping

¼ cup cilantro leaves, for topping

1. Heat oil in a large saucepan on medium. Add yellow onion and cook, stirring occasionally, 3 to 5 minutes. Stir in garlic and ginger; cook 1 minute.

2. Add guava paste, vinegar, rum, tomato paste, soy sauce, Worcestershire, ½ cup water, and ½ teaspoon salt; simmer, stirring often, until slightly thickened, 5 to 6 minutes. Transfer to a blender and puree until smooth. Return to saucepan, add jackfruit and ½ cup water, and barely simmer, covered, 15 minutes.

3. Stir and continue cooking until jackfruit is very tender, adding water if mixture seems too thick, 10 to 12 minutes more. Using a potato masher, shred jackfruit until it resembles pulled pork.

4. Meanwhile, in a small bowl, toss jalapeño, red onion, lime juice, and remaining ¼ teaspoon salt. Let sit at least 5 minutes.

5. Serve jackfruit on buns, topped with pickled jalapeño, red onion, avocado, and cilantro.

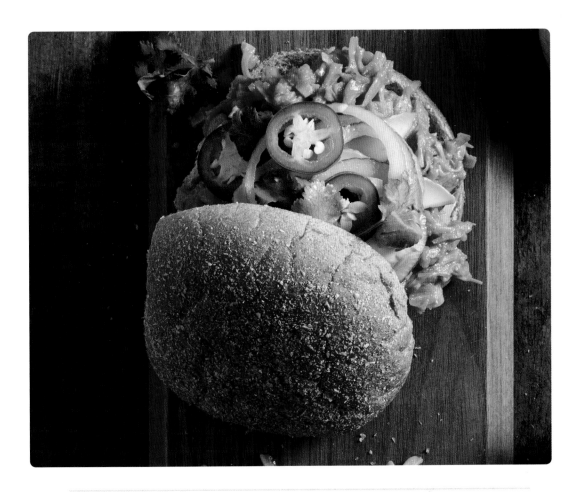

PER SERVING 475 calories, 13.5 g fat (2 g saturated fat), 11 g protein, 740 mg sodium, 78 g carbohydrates, 22 g fiber, 35 g sugars (29.5 g added sugars), 0 mg cholesterol

TIP Jackfruit, a trendy meat alternative, is a real fruit, so you can buy it fresh, crack it open, and use the tender flesh inside. For an easier option, you can find it packaged (try Upton's Naturals' Original flavor). Jackfruit is high in protein and fiber, has a soft texture, and takes on the flavor of what you cook it with, making it great in sauce-heavy dishes, stews, curries, and—in perhaps its most popular use—faux BBQ pulled pork, as shown here.

"B"LT

Tempeh has long been used as a substitute for bacon—and for good reason: It closely mimics that familiar sweet, smoky flavor. It also has a contribution to make toward lowering cholesterol and improving bone health.

1 (6-ounce) block tempeh, sliced into bacon-like pieces

1 tablespoon soy sauce

1 teaspoon liquid smoke

1 tablespoon canola oil

1 tablespoon mayonnaise

2 teaspoons hot sauce, (such as sriracha)

4 slices sourdough bread, toasted

½ avocado

1 tomato, thinly sliced

2 leaves romaine lettuce

1. In a large resealable plastic bag, combine tempeh, soy sauce, and liquid smoke. Refrigerate for at least 1 hour or up to 4 hours.

2. Heat oil in a pan on medium-high. Add tempeh and sear until browned, 1 to 2 minutes per side. Transfer to a plate.

3. In a small bowl, mix mayonnaise and hot sauce. Slather 1 side of 2 slices of bread with spicy mayo. Mash half the avocado into 1 side of the other 2 bread slices. Layer each sandwich with tempeh, tomato, and lettuce. Close sandwiches before serving.

PER SERVING 555 calories, 30 g fat (5 g saturated fat), 27 g protein, 1,015 mg sodium, 50 g carbohydrates, 3 g fiber, 5 g sugars (0 g added sugars), 3 mg cholesterol

SPICED TOFU TACOS 🌱

TOTAL TIME: 20 MINUTES ◆ SERVES 4

These weeknight treats are packed with filling protein from the tofu. To keep your tofu from being too soggy, wrap the block in paper towels, place it on a plate, and set another plate on top of it to press out more of the water.

½ small poblano chile

½ red pepper

2 cloves garlic

1 small onion

1 tablespoon oil

1 package extra-firm tofu, squeezed of excess moisture

1½ teaspoons chili powder

½ teaspoon ground coriander

¼ teaspoon salt

¼ teaspoon black pepper

8 corn tortillas

Romaine lettuce, shredded, for topping

1 jalapeño, sliced, for topping

1. In a food processor, finely chop chile, red pepper, garlic, and onion. In a large nonstick skillet, cook mixture in oil, stirring occasionally, 4 minutes.

2. Crumble tofu into the skillet and season with chili powder, coriander, salt, and black pepper; cook, stirring occasionally, until golden brown.

3. Spoon into tortillas; top with lettuce and jalapeños.

PER SERVING 230 calories, 10 g fat (1 g saturated fat), 13 g protein, 170 mg sodium, 24 g carbohydrates, 6 g fiber, 5 g sugars (0 g added sugars), 0 mg cholesterol

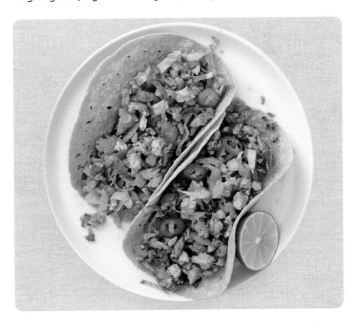

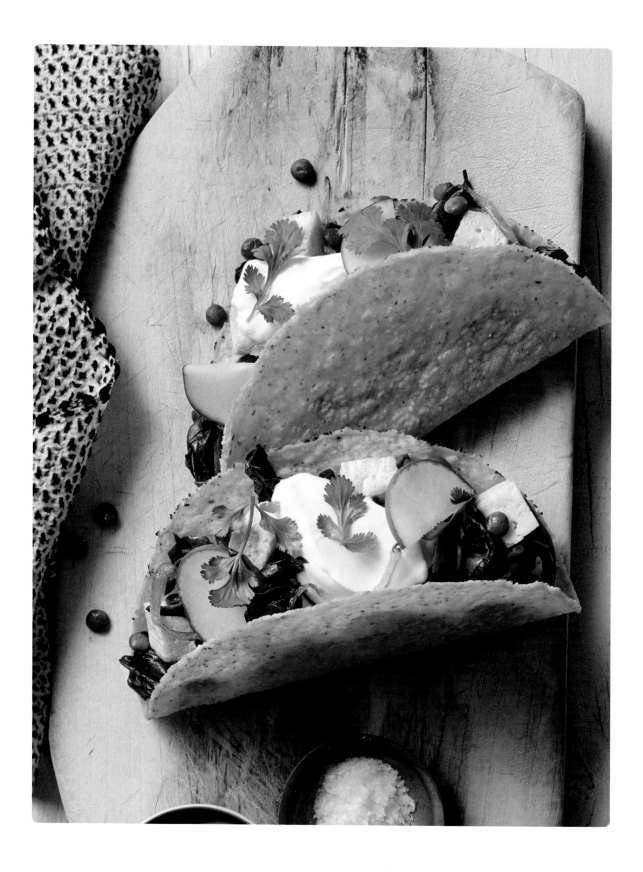

TOFU, LENTIL & SWISS CHARD TACOS

TOTAL TIME: 30 MINUTES ◆ SERVES 4

Swiss chard is a leafy green with a subtly bitter bite that mellows slightly when cooked. It's a good source of vitamins A (for eye health), C (for tissue repair) and K (to build bones).

3 tablespoons vegetable oil, divided

1 (12-ounce) package extra-firm tofu, pressed and cut into ½-inch cubes

Kosher salt

Black pepper

½ large onion, sliced

1 large chipotle chile in adobo, chopped, plus 2 tablespoons adobo sauce

1 (15-ounce) can lentils, drained and rinsed

4 cups chopped Swiss chard

8 corn taco shells

¼ cup plain fat-free Greek yogurt

Sliced radishes, for topping

Cilantro leaves, for topping

Lime wedges, for serving

1. Heat 2 tablespoons oil in a large skillet on medium-high. Season tofu with salt and pepper to taste and cook until golden, about 6 minutes. Transfer tofu to a paper-towel-lined plate.

2. Heat remaining 1 tablespoon oil in the skillet and add onion. Cook until soft, about 5 minutes. Add chile, adobo sauce, lentils, and chard; cook until chard wilts, about 4 minutes.

3. Return tofu to pan, toss to combine, and season with salt and pepper to taste. Divide mixture among taco shells. Top with yogurt, radishes, and cilantro. Serve with lime wedges.

PER SERVING 465 calories, 22 g fat (2.5 g saturated fat), 22 g protein, 435 mg sodium, 49 g carbohydrates, 13 g fiber, 6 g sugars (0 g added sugars), 435 mg cholesterol

SWEET & STICKY TOFU 🌱

TOTAL TIME: 30 MINUTES ◆ SERVES 4

When you don't get enough iron in your diet, you may end up feeling perpetually sluggish. Bok choy's vitamin C helps you absorb tofu's iron more effectively, assisting in transporting oxygen throughout your body.

4 ounces udon noodles

2 tablespoons reduced-sodium soy sauce

1 teaspoon brown sugar

1 teaspoon cornstarch

½ teaspoon black pepper

14 ounces firm tofu, drained

2 tablespoons canola oil, divided

2 cloves garlic, finely chopped

1 (1-inch) piece ginger, peeled and cut into matchsticks

4 scallions, thinly sliced

1 small red chile, thinly sliced

2 bunches baby bok choy, leaves separated and halved lengthwise

2 cups baby spinach

1. Cook noodles per package directions. In a small bowl, combine ¼ cup water, soy sauce, brown sugar, cornstarch, and ½ teaspoon pepper until smooth.

2. Blot tofu dry with paper towels. Cut into ¾-inch pieces. Heat a large skillet on medium-high. Add 1 tablespoon oil, then tofu, and cook, stirring occasionally, until golden brown, 6 to 8 minutes. Transfer to a plate; wipe out skillet.

3. Add remaining 1 tablespoon oil, then garlic, ginger, half the scallions, and chile; cook 1 minute. Add bok choy and cook, tossing, 2 minutes.

4. Fold in tofu, then soy sauce mixture. Simmer until thickened, about 1 minute; toss with spinach. Spoon over noodles and top with remaining scallions and chile.

PER SERVING 270 calories, 12 g fat (1 g saturated fat), 15 g protein, 405 mg sodium, 27 g carbohydrates, 5 g fiber, 3 g sugars (1 g added sugars), 0 mg cholesterol

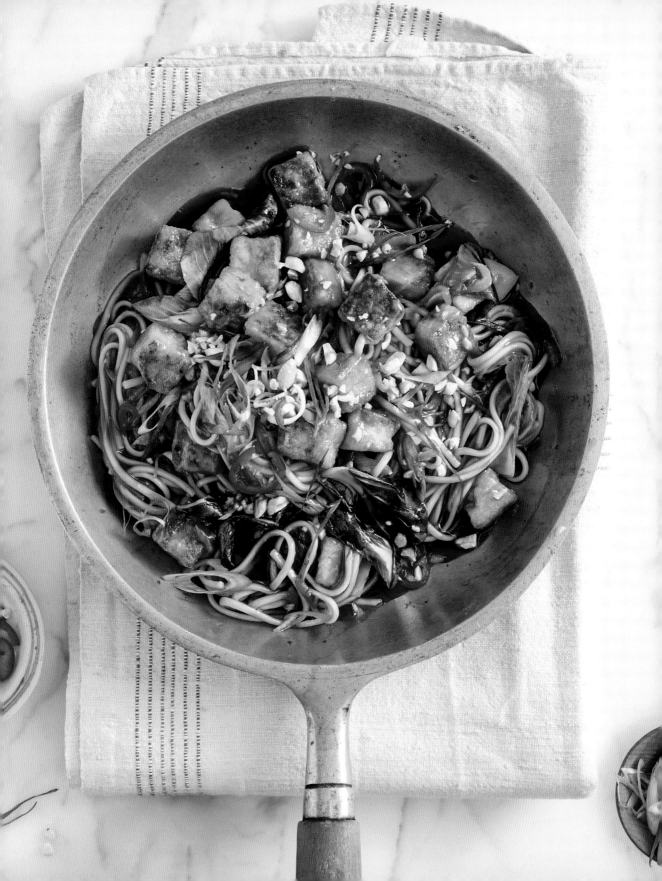

ASIAN TOFU WITH BABY BOK CHOY

TOTAL TIME: 1 HOUR ◆ **SERVES 4**

This one-dish wonder is brimming with flavor and good-for-you ingredients. Assemble all ingredients on a baking sheet, pop it in the oven, and it will be ready in 30 minutes—it's as easy as that.

1 (14-ounce) block extra-firm tofu

4 teaspoons low-sodium soy sauce

1 tablespoon chili-garlic sauce

1 clove garlic, pressed

1 teaspoon honey

6 teaspoons toasted sesame oil, divided

Vegetable oil, for the baking sheet

8 small bunches baby bok choy, trimmed and halved lengthwise

4 sugar snap peas, thinly sliced

½ teaspoon black sesame seeds

1. Place tofu on a rimmed baking sheet between paper towels. Top with another baking sheet and weigh down with heavy cans or a skillet; let sit 30 minutes.

2. Meanwhile, in a small bowl, combine soy sauce, chili-garlic sauce, garlic, honey, and 4 teaspoons sesame oil.

3. Heat oven to 400°F. Transfer tofu to a cutting board. Wipe off the baking sheet and lightly oil. Slice tofu into ½-inch-thick triangles and arrange on prepared sheet. Drizzle with 1 tablespoon sauce mixture and bake until top is golden, 12 to 15 minutes.

4. Turn tofu over, arrange on one side of the baking sheet, and drizzle with 1 tablespoon sauce mixture. Arrange bok choy on other half of the sheet and gently toss with remaining 2 teaspoons sesame oil.

5. Roast until tofu is golden brown and bok choy is tender, 8 to 12 minutes more. Drizzle remaining sauce over tofu and sprinkle everything with sugar snap peas and sesame seeds.

PER SERVING 195 calories, 12.5 g fat (1.5 g saturated fat), 13 g protein, 380 mg sodium, 10 g carbohydrates, 4 g fiber, 5 g sugars (2 g added sugars), 0 mg cholesterol

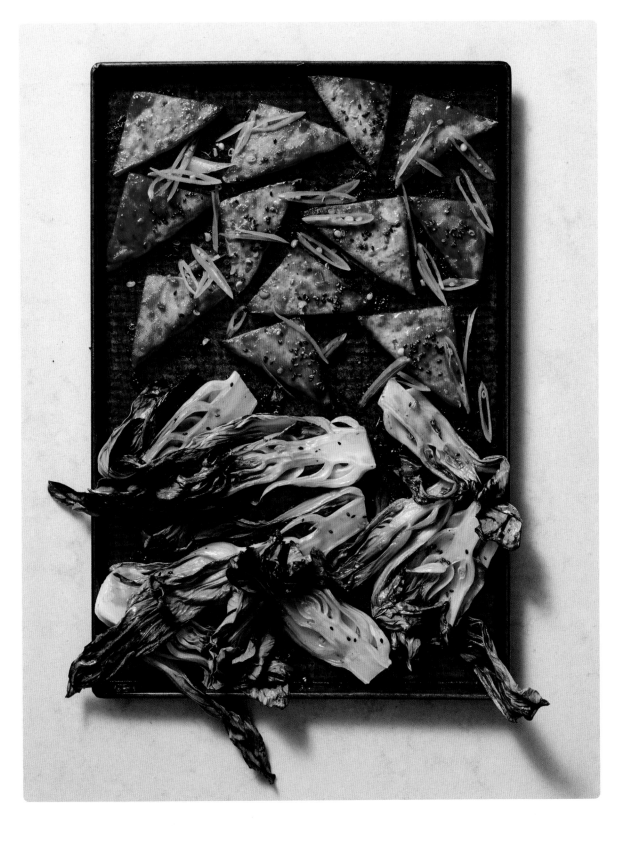

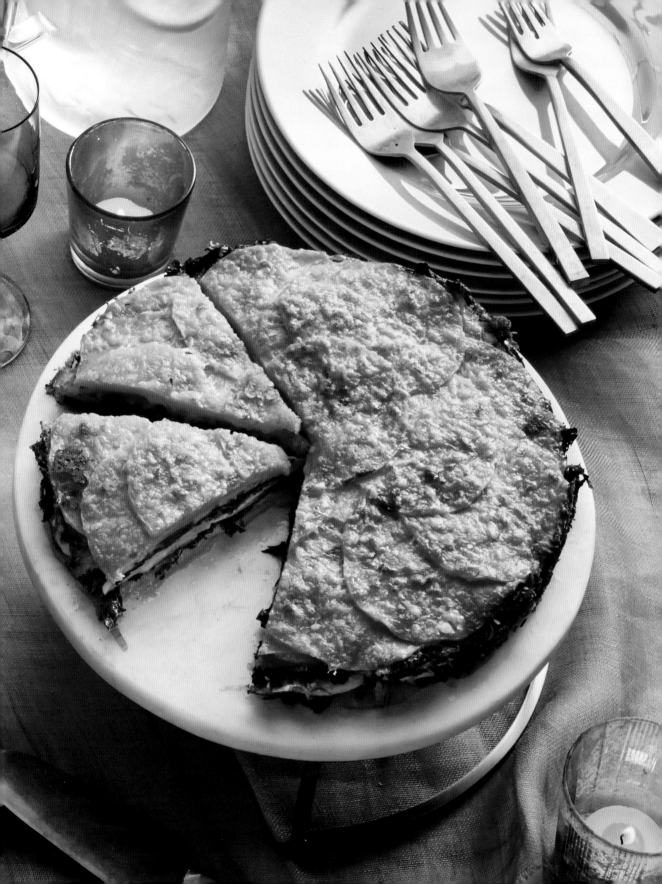

BUTTERNUT SQUASH & KALE TORTE

TOTAL TIME: 45 MINUTES ◆ SERVES 8

This is how plant-based fare should taste: layered like lasagna with flavorful vegetables and nutty cheese. If the torte feels too fancy, prepare it casserole style in a baking dish and serve by scooping out portions.

1 tablespoon olive oil, divided, plus more for the pan

½ small butternut squash (about 1 pound), peeled and thinly sliced

1 red onion, thinly sliced

1 small bunch kale, thick stems discarded and leaves cut into 1-inch pieces

½ teaspoon kosher salt, divided

¼ teaspoon black pepper

1 medium yellow potato, thinly sliced

4 ounces sharp provolone cheese, thinly sliced

1 plum tomato, thinly sliced

1 ounce Parmesan cheese, grated (about ¼ cup)

1. Heat oven to 425°F. Oil a 9-inch springform pan. Arrange half the squash in concentric circles in the bottom of the pan. Top with half the onion, then half the kale. Drizzle with ½ tablespoon oil and season with ¼ teaspoon salt. Top with potato and half the provolone.

2. Top with remaining kale, drizzle with remaining ½ tablespoon oil, and season with ¼ teaspoon each salt and pepper. Top with remaining onion, tomato, and remaining provolone. Arrange remaining squash on top and sprinkle with Parmesan.

3. Cover with foil, place on a baking sheet, and bake 20 minutes. Uncover and bake until tender and top is browned, 8 to 10 minutes.

PER SERVING 140 calories, 7 g fat (3.5 g saturated fat), 7 g protein, 305 mg sodium, 14 g carbohydrates, 2 g fiber, 2.5 g sugars (0 g added sugars), 12 mg cholesterol

TIP Remove kale stems quickly with this easy method: Fold the leaf in half lengthwise, exposing the stem in the back. Using a sharp knife, cut away the stem.

ROASTED TOMATO & EGGPLANT TACOS ✿

TOTAL TIME: 30 MINUTES ◆ SERVES 4

Eggplant's anthocyanins, the compounds that give the vegetable its deep violet hue, may protect your brain against aging, so eat up!

10 ounces cherry tomatoes

½ pound eggplant, cut into ½-inch chunks

2 tablespoons olive oil

1 teaspoon ground cumin

¼ teaspoon allspice

1 large yellow onion, thinly sliced

¾ teaspoon kosher salt, divided

¾ teaspoon black pepper, divided

¼ cup tahini

1 tablespoon lemon juice

8 blue corn taco shells

Mint leaves, for serving

1. Heat oven to 450°F. On a baking sheet, toss tomatoes, eggplant, oil, cumin, allspice, onion, and ½ teaspoon each salt and pepper. Roast until veggies are tender, about 12 minutes.

2. In a bowl, whisk together tahini, lemon juice, 2 to 4 tablespoons water, and remaining ¼ teaspoon each salt and pepper.

3. Serve veggies in taco shells, topped with tahini and mint.

PER SERVING 290 calories, 19.5 g fat (3 g saturated fat), 6 g protein, 460 mg sodium, 26 g carbohydrates, 5 g fiber, 5 g sugars (0 g added sugars), 0 mg cholesterol

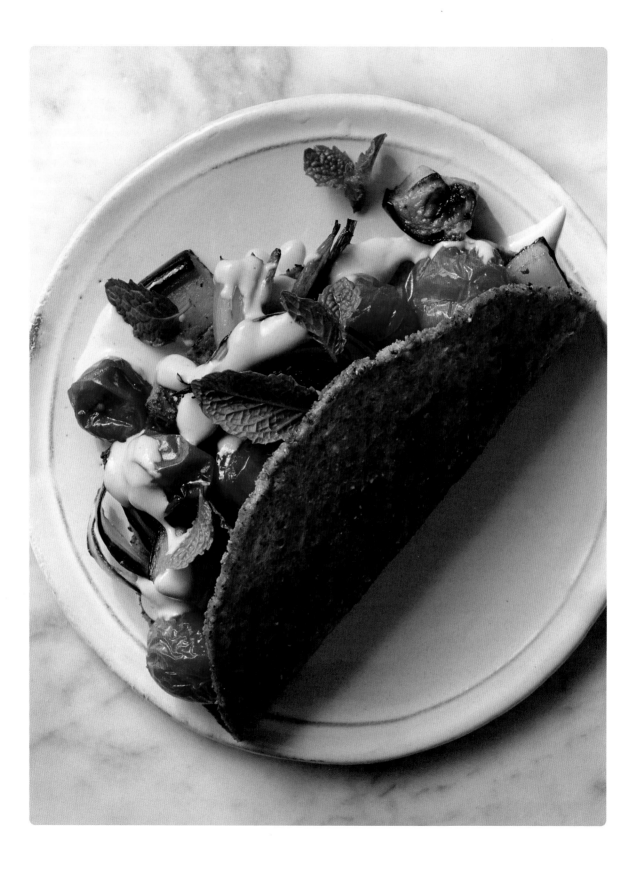

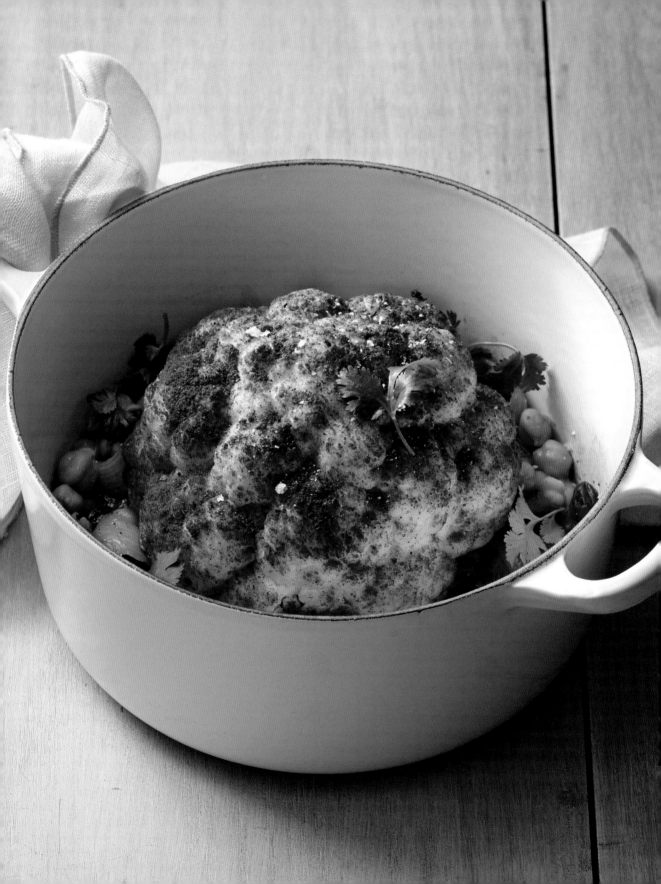

MOROCCAN CAULIFLOWER POT ROAST ❧

You won't miss the meat once you taste this hearty, flavorful cauliflower enhanced with deep, rich spices. This one-dish delight includes nutty, satisfying chickpeas and surprisingly savory raisins to round out the dinner menu.

2 teaspoons ground coriander

1½ teaspoons ground cumin

1½ teaspoons chili powder

1 teaspoon turmeric

¾ teaspoon sugar

½ teaspoon cinnamon

½ teaspoon kosher salt

½ teaspoon black pepper

1 large head cauliflower

3 teaspoons olive oil, divided

1 onion, sliced into ½-inch wedges

1 clove garlic, sliced

1 (15-ounce) can chickpeas, drained and rinsed

3 tablespoons raisins

2 cups reduced-sodium vegetable broth

1. Heat oven to 375°F. In a bowl, combine coriander, cumin, chili powder, turmeric, sugar, cinnamon, salt, and pepper.

2. Slice stalk from cauliflower so it sits flat; score bottom with an X. Brush with 1½ teaspoons oil; coat with spice rub. Heat remaining 1½ teaspoons oil in a heavy pot on medium. Add onion and garlic; cook until onion begins to soften, 5 minutes. Add chickpeas and raisins; cook 3 minutes more.
Add broth, bring to a simmer, and place cauliflower into pot, spice side up.

3. Cover and bake 30 minutes. Remove cover; continue baking until cauliflower is tender, 25 to 30 minutes more. Slice cauliflower into wedges and serve with chickpea mix and liquid.

PER SERVING 135 calories, 4 g fat (0.5 g saturated fat), 6 g protein, 380 mg sodium, 22 g carbohydrates, 6 g fiber, 7 g sugars (0 g added sugars), 0 mg cholesterol

GREEK STUFFED TOMATOES

TOTAL TIME: 2 HOURS ◆ SERVES 10

To make preparing this dish a snap, use the grating blade on a food processor to prep the vegetables for the stuffing.

10 large tomatoes

2 zucchini, grated

1 onion, grated

1 potato, grated

¼ cup short-grain brown rice

¼ cup chopped flat-leaf parsley

2 tablespoons finely chopped mint

1 tablespoon finely chopped oregano

3 garlic cloves, minced

½ cup olive oil, divided

¼ cup lemon juice

1 teaspoon kosher salt

½ teaspoon black pepper

1 cup plain low-fat Greek yogurt

1. Heat oven to 400°F. Use a serrated knife to slice ¼ inch from top of each tomato; set aside. Using spoon, scoop out tomato flesh, and coarsely chop. Transfer to a large bowl. Arrange tomatoes in a large baking dish.

2. To the large bowl with tomato flesh, stir in zucchini, onion, potato, rice, parsley, mint, oregano, and garlic. Add ¼ cup oil, lemon juice, salt, and pepper, and mix thoroughly.

3. Divide filling among all tomatoes, place tops on them, and drizzle with remaining ¼ cup oil. Pour 1 cup water into the baking dish and bake 20 minutes.

4. Reduce oven temperature to 325°F. Cover dish with foil, and continue baking until rice is cooked through, about 1 hour, adding more water if the baking dish dries out.

5. Remove from oven. Remove foil, and let tomatoes sit 10 minutes. Dollop with yogurt before serving.

PER SERVING 225 calories, 12 g fat (2 g saturated fat), 6 g protein, 215 mg sodium, 26 g carbohydrates, 4 g fiber, 7 g sugars (0 g added sugars), 0 mg cholesterol

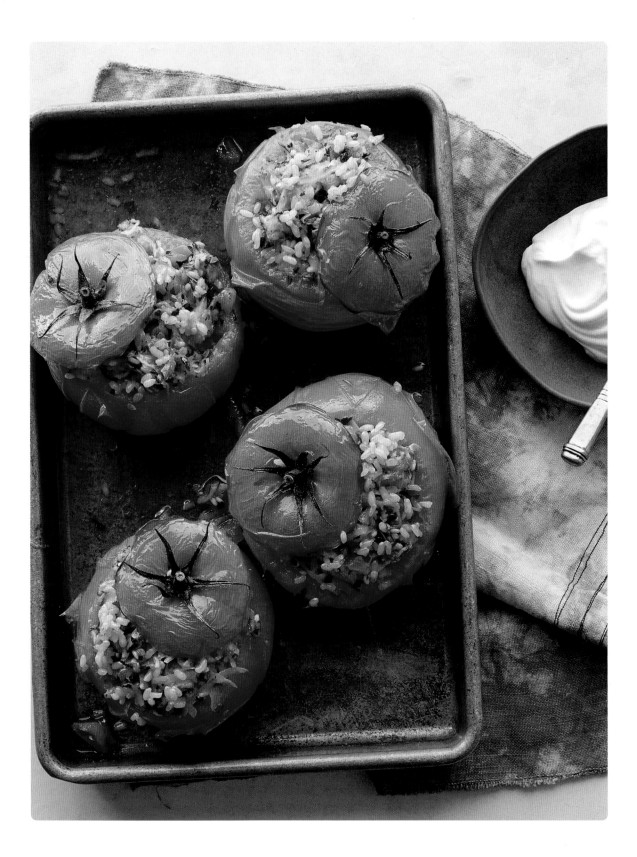

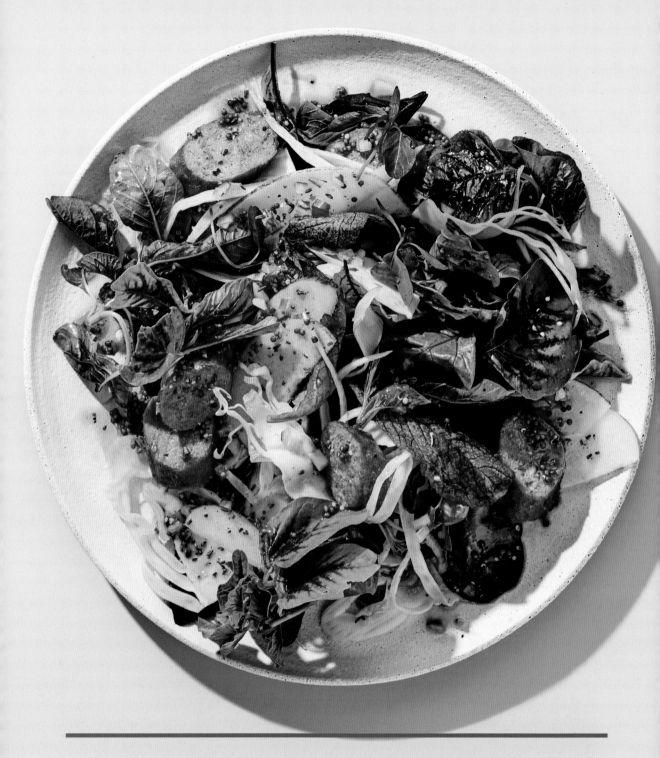

TIP If you can't find vegan bratwurst, you can substitute any other kind of vegan meat—or, if you're really in the mood, the real thing. Plant-based eating is all about balance!

VEGAN BRATWURST & APPLE SALAD
WITH CARAWAY VINAIGRETTE ❧

TOTAL TIME: 20 MINUTES ◆ SERVES 4

The sausage in this recipe is not actually meat, but you won't notice the difference. When you're cooking, make sure you leave the peel on your apple—about half of the fruit's fiber is found in the skin.

1 teaspoon caraway seeds, crushed

3 tablespoons sherry vinegar

1 tablespoon whole-grain mustard

⅛ teaspoon kosher salt

⅛ teaspoon black pepper

½ small red onion, finely chopped

4 vegan bratwursts (about 12 ounces)

2 tablespoons olive oil

1 small fennel bulb, cored and thinly sliced

1 Gala apple, thinly sliced

6 cups mixed greens

1. Heat a small pan on medium and toast caraway seeds until fragrant, about 2 minutes. In a large bowl, whisk together vinegar, mustard, salt, and pepper. Mix in caraway, then onion; let sit 5 minutes.

2. Meanwhile, cook sausages per package directions, then slice.

3. Toss onion mixture with oil, then add fennel and apple. Fold in greens and sausage.

PER SERVING 335 calories, 20.5 g fat (6.5 g saturated fat), 20 g protein, 710 mg sodium, 19 g carbohydrates, 7 g fiber, 8 g sugars (0.5 g added sugars), 0 mg cholesterol

EASY TEMPEH LETTUCE WRAPS

TOTAL TIME: 10 MINUTES ◆ SERVES 1

When cooked correctly, tempeh is one of the most meat-like alternatives to animal proteins. Pairing it with heart-healthy zucchini and immune-boosting red cabbage, these wraps combine great flavor with satisfying crunch.

½ cup cooked quinoa

¼ cup chopped zucchini

¼ cup chopped onions

¼ cup chopped tomatoes

Coarse salt

Black pepper

3 leaves Boston lettuce

1 piece roasted tempeh, chopped

¼ cup shredded red cabbage

Cilantro or mint leaves

2 tablespoons plain 2-percent Greek yogurt

Lime wedges, for serving

1. Toss cooked quinoa with chopped zucchini, onions, and tomatoes. Season with a pinch of coarse salt and pepper to taste.

2. Fill lettuce leaves with quinoa-vegetable mixture and top with chopped tempeh, shredded red cabbage, cilantro or mint, and Greek yogurt to make 3 taco-like wraps. Serve with lime wedges.

PER SERVING 395 calories, 16 g fat (5 g saturated fat), 32 g protein, 160 mg sodium, 39 g carbohydrates, 5 g fiber, 6 g sugars (0 g added sugars), 3 mg cholesterol

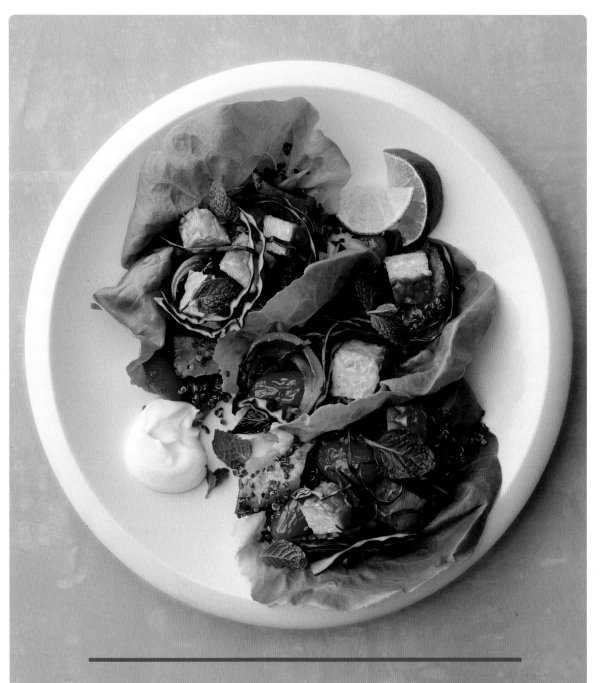

TIP Haven't heard of tempeh? It's made from soybeans just like tofu, but it is firmer, has a nutty flavor, and is packed with protein, vitamins, and minerals.

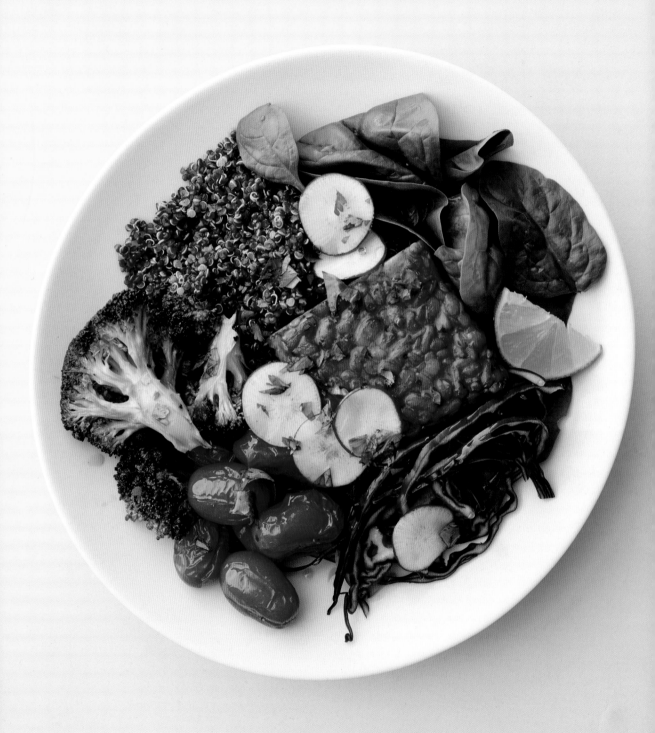

ROASTED VEGGIE & TEMPEH BOWL 🌱

TOTAL TIME: 30 MINUTES ◆ **SERVES 1**

This meal is versatile: Swap chicken for the tempeh, cooked farro for the quinoa, and kale for the spinach. And lemon juice or even grapefruit juice works just as well as lime. You could even garnish with scallions or snow peas instead of radishes.

1 (8-ounce) package tempeh

¼ cup reduced-sodium tamari

3 tablespoons olive oil

2 tablespoons lime juice

6 cloves garlic

1 tablespoons peeled and grated ginger

1 cup baby spinach

½ cup shredded red cabbage

½ cup cooked quinoa

1 cup leftover roasted veggies (such as ½ cup each grape tomatoes and broccoli)

2 tablespoons chopped cilantro

¼ teaspoon toasted sesame oil

Sliced radishes, for topping

Lime wedge, for serving

1. Heat oven to 425°F. Cut the tempeh crosswise into 2 pieces and place in a foil-lined baking pan.

2. In a small bowl, whisk together tamari, olive oil, lime juice, garlic, and ginger; spoon over tempeh and turn to coat. Place in the pan and roast until golden brown, 12 to 15 minutes. Let cool.

3. In a large bowl, combine spinach, cabbage, quinoa, roasted vegetables, and 1 piece of tempeh. (Refrigerate remaining tempeh in an airtight container for another use.) Sprinkle with cilantro and drizzle with sesame oil. Top with sliced radishes and serve with lime wedge.

PER SERVING 640 calories, 36 g fat (6 g saturated fat), 36 g protein, 1,500 mg sodium, 50 g carbohydrates, 9 g fiber, 5 g sugars (0 g added sugars), 0 mg cholesterol

BUTTERNUT SQUASH & MOLE ENCHILADAS

TOTAL TIME: 1 HOUR ◆ SERVES 6

Mole, a traditional Mexican sauce, transforms niacin-rich butternut squash into these cholesterol-lowering, vegetarian enchiladas. To make them vegan, just skip the queso.

2 pounds butternut squash, peeled and cut into ½-inch pieces

1 tablespoon olive oil

¼ teaspoon chili powder

Pinch plus ¼ teaspoon kosher salt

Pinch plus ¼ teaspoon black pepper

1 (15-ounce) can tomato sauce

2 cloves garlic

½ small onion, chopped

1 chipotle chile in adobo, plus 1 tablespoon adobo sauce

½ teaspoon cinnamon

1 tablespoon lime juice

¼ cup smooth peanut butter

3 ounces semisweet chocolate

Cooking spray

12 soft corn tortillas

1 (15-ounce) can black beans, drained and rinsed

4 ounces queso fresco, crumbled, plus more for topping

1 avocado, cut into chunks, for topping

Toasted pepitas for topping

Cilantro leaves, for serving

1. Heat oven to 400°F. On a rimmed baking sheet, toss squash with oil, chili powder, and a pinch each salt and pepper. Roast until tender, 15 to 20 minutes. Set aside. Lower oven to 350°F.

2. Meanwhile, make mole: In blender, puree tomato sauce, garlic, onion, chile, adobo sauce, cinnamon, lime juice, and remaining ¼ teaspoon each salt and pepper until smooth. Transfer to small saucepan and simmer on medium, 4 minutes. Add peanut butter and chocolate, stirring until smooth. Remove from heat.

3. Coat a 9- by 13-inch baking dish with cooking spray, then spread a third of mole sauce on bottom. Fill each tortilla with scant ¼ cup squash and 1 tablespoon each black beans and queso fresco. Roll and place seam side down in prepared dish.

4. Spoon another ¼ of mole over top, cover, and bake 20 minutes. Uncover, spread with remaining mole, and bake 5 minutes more. Remove from oven and top with queso fresco, avocado, pepitas, and cilantro.

PER SERVING 490 calories, 25 g fat (8 g saturated fat), 15 g protein, 865 mg sodium, 60 g carbohydrates, 13 g fiber, 18 g sugars (8 g added sugars), 20 mg cholesterol

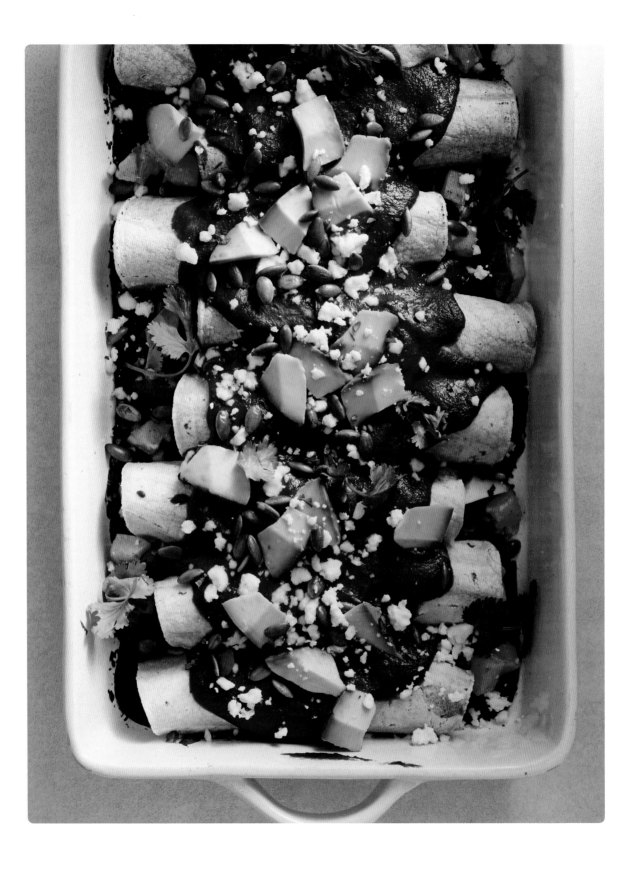

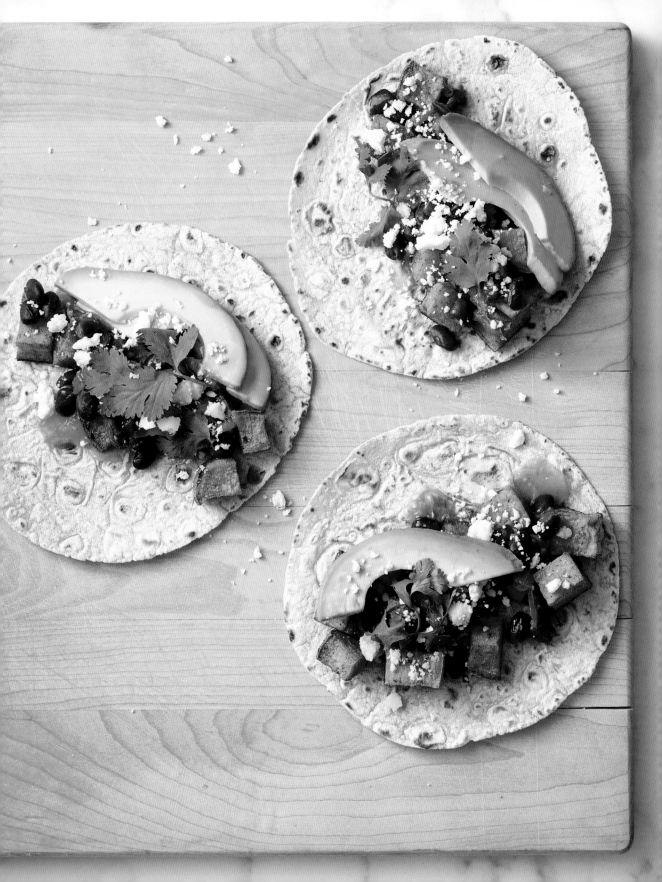

SWEET POTATO, AVOCADO & BLACK BEAN TACOS

TOTAL TIME: 40 MINUTES ♦ SERVES 4

Corn tortillas are lower in carbohydrates, fat, and calories than their flour counterparts, and they're actually considered a whole grain.

1¾ pounds sweet potatoes, scrubbed and cut into ½-inch chunks

1 tablespoon olive oil

1 teaspoon chili powder

Kosher salt

1 (15-ounce) can no-salt-added black beans, drained and rinsed

½ cup salsa verde

1 avocado, thinly sliced

8 corn tortillas

¼ cup crumbled Cotija or feta cheese

Cilantro leaves, for topping

1. Heat oven to 450°F. Toss sweet potatoes with oil, chili powder, and salt to taste. Arrange on a large rimmed baking sheet; roast 30 minutes.

2. In a saucepan on medium, combine black beans with salsa verde; cook, stirring, until warm.

3. Serve sweet potatoes and beans with avocado, corn tortillas, cheese, and cilantro.

PER SERVING 465 calories, 16 g fat (3 g saturated fat), 13 g protein, 715 mg sodium, 70 g carbohydrates, 16 g fiber, 12 g sugars (0 g added sugars), 6 mg cholesterol

LENTIL-BROCCOLI FALAFEL BOWL WITH JALAPEÑO-HERB TAHINI

TOTAL TIME: 1 HOUR ◆ SERVES 6

Nothing goes to waste in this veggie-packed dinner—even the cilantro stems find a home in the zesty tahini sauce. Even better, this recipe comes out to less than five dollars per serving.

1 jalapeño, halved lengthwise, seeded

2 teaspoons plus 5 tablespoons olive oil, divided

1 cup brown rice

2 small sweet potatoes, cut into 1-inch wedges

Kosher salt

Black pepper

¼ medium onion, roughly chopped

1 pound broccoli, stems sliced, tops cut into florets, separated

1 pound cremini mushrooms

1 bunch cilantro

¼ cup tahini

6 tablespoons lemon juice, divided

1 clove garlic, chopped

5 ounces cooked (or canned) lentils, rinsed

2 teaspoons lemon zest

1½ teaspoons paprika

1 teaspoon ground cumin

½ teaspoon ground coriander

½ teaspoon dried oregano

½ teaspoon ground fennel seed

1 large egg

4 cups kale leaves, torn into small pieces

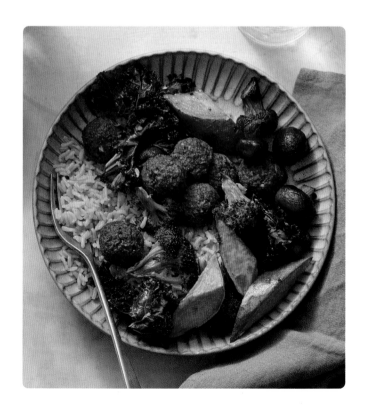

1. Heat broiler. On a small baking sheet, toss jalapeño with 2 teaspoons oil and broil until charred, 3 minutes per side; let cool.

2. Reduce oven temp to 425°F. Cook rice per package directions. On a rimmed baking sheet, toss sweet potatoes with 1 tablespoon oil, salt, and pepper. On a second baking sheet, toss onion, 6 ounces broccoli stems, and 4 ounces mushrooms with 1 tablespoon oil; arrange on one side of the pan. On other side, toss remaining broccoli and mushrooms with 1 tablespoon oil and ¼ teaspoon pepper. Roast both pans until vegetables are golden brown and tender, 15 to 20 minutes for broccoli and 25 to 30 minutes for sweet potatoes.

3. While vegetables are roasting, prepare sauce: Bring a pot of water to a boil and fill a large bowl with ice water. Dip cilantro in boiling water for 30 seconds, then transfer to ice bath. Once cool, squeeze as much excess water from cilantro as possible, then roughly chop. Transfer to a blender along with charred jalapeño, tahini, 2 tablespoons lemon juice, ⅓ cup water, and ¼ teaspoon salt; puree until mostly smooth, about 1 minute. Set aside.

4. Make the falafel: Place roasted-onion mixture in a food processor with garlic, lentils, lemon zest, 2 tablespoons lemon juice, spices, and ½ teaspoon salt; pulse to combine. Add egg and pulse to combine. Form 18 heaping tablespoon-size balls, transfer to a parchment-lined baking sheet, and roast until golden brown, 10 to 12 minutes.

5. Meanwhile, in a bowl, toss kale with remaining 2 tablespoons each lemon juice and oil and a pinch of salt. Divide rice among bowls. Top with sweet potatoes, broccoli and mushrooms, kale leaves, and falafel. Serve drizzled with jalapeño-herb tahini.

PER SERVING 425 calories, 20.5 g fat (3 g saturated fat), 14 g protein, 375 mg sodium, 48 g carbohydrates, 10 g fiber, 6 g sugars (0 g added sugars), 30 mg cholesterol

"FRIED" AVOCADO TACOS

TOTAL TIME: 40 MINUTES ◆ SERVES 8

Take the buttery flavor (and healthy fats) of avocado to the next level by rolling slices in breadcrumbs and baking them to crispy perfection. Then use as the filling for these craveable tacos.

¼ cup all-purpose flour

¼ teaspoon plus a pinch kosher salt

¼ teaspoon black pepper

2 large egg whites

1 cup panko breadcrumbs

2 tablespoons olive oil

2 medium firm but ripe avocados

1 lime, plus wedges for serving

4 tablespoons mayonnaise

½ small red cabbage (about 1 pound), cored and thinly sliced

2 scallions, thinly sliced

1 jalapeño, seeded and thinly sliced

½ cup cilantro leaves, plus more for serving

8 small flour tortillas, warmed

Sour cream, for serving

1. Heat oven to 425°F. Line a large rimmed baking sheet with nonstick foil.

2. In a small bowl, whisk together flour, ¼ teaspoon salt, and pepper. In a second small bowl, lightly beat egg whites. In a third small bowl, combine panko with oil.

3. Cut avocados in half; remove pit and peel. Cut each half into ½-inch slices. Working with one slice at a time, lightly coat avocado slices in flour, then in egg, letting any excess drip off, and finally in panko, pressing gently to help it adhere. Transfer to the baking sheet and repeat with remaining slices. Bake until golden brown, 20 to 25 minutes.

4. Meanwhile, finely grate lime zest into a large bowl, then squeeze in 2 tablespoons lime juice. Whisk in mayonnaise and remaining pinch of salt. Add cabbage, scallions, and jalapeño, and toss to coat; fold in cilantro. Fill tortillas with avocado slices and top with cabbage slaw. Serve with extra cilantro, lime wedges, and sour cream, if desired.

PER SERVING 650 calories, 35 g fat (6 g saturated fat), 4 g protein, 910 mg sodium, 72 g carbohydrates, 12 g fiber, 7 g sugars (0 g added sugars), 5 mg cholesterol

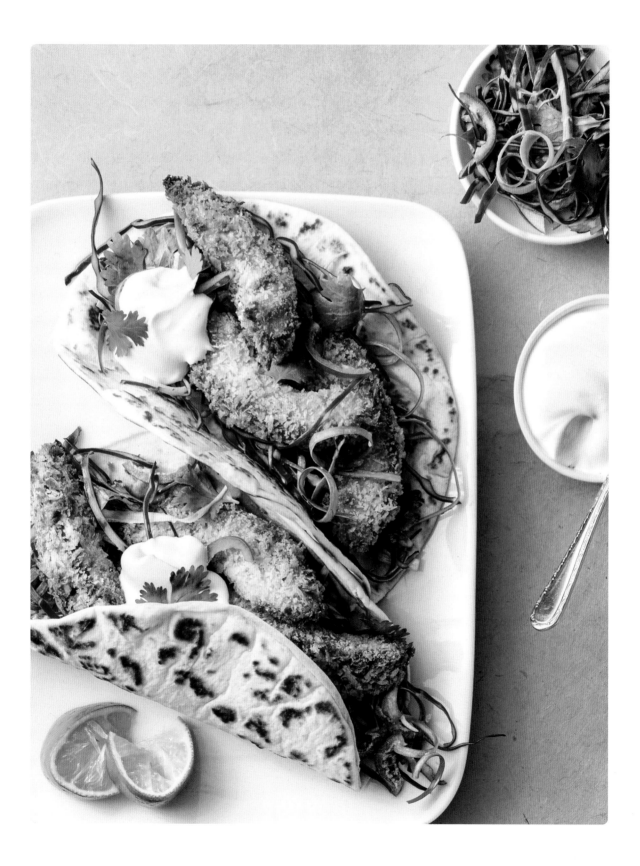

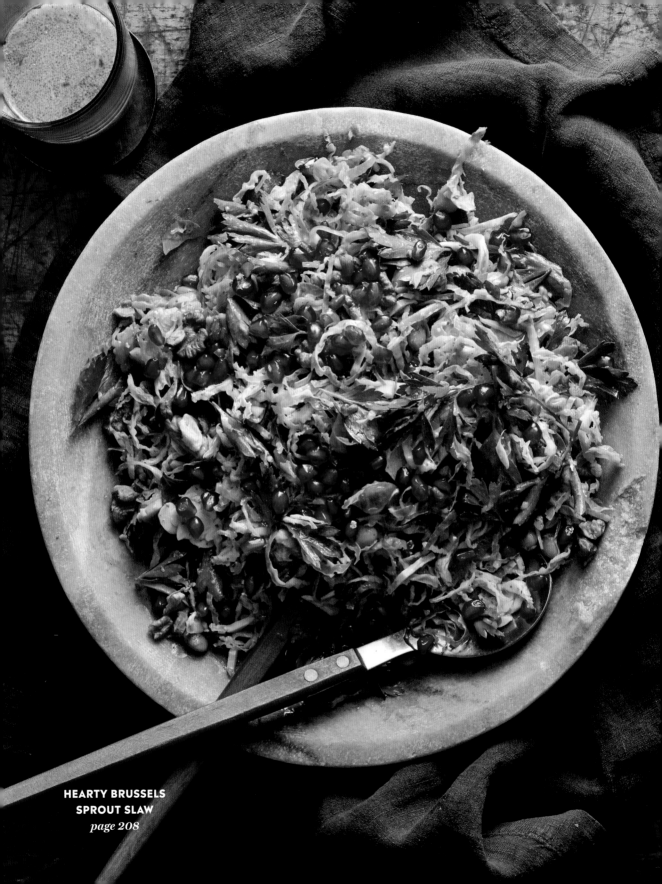

**HEARTY BRUSSELS
SPROUT SLAW**
page 208

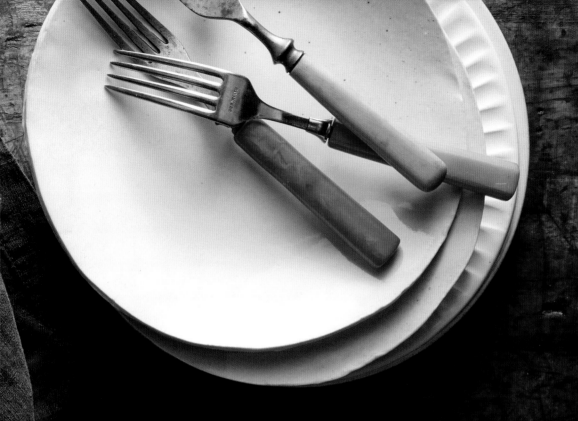

Chapter 5

SIDES & SNACKS

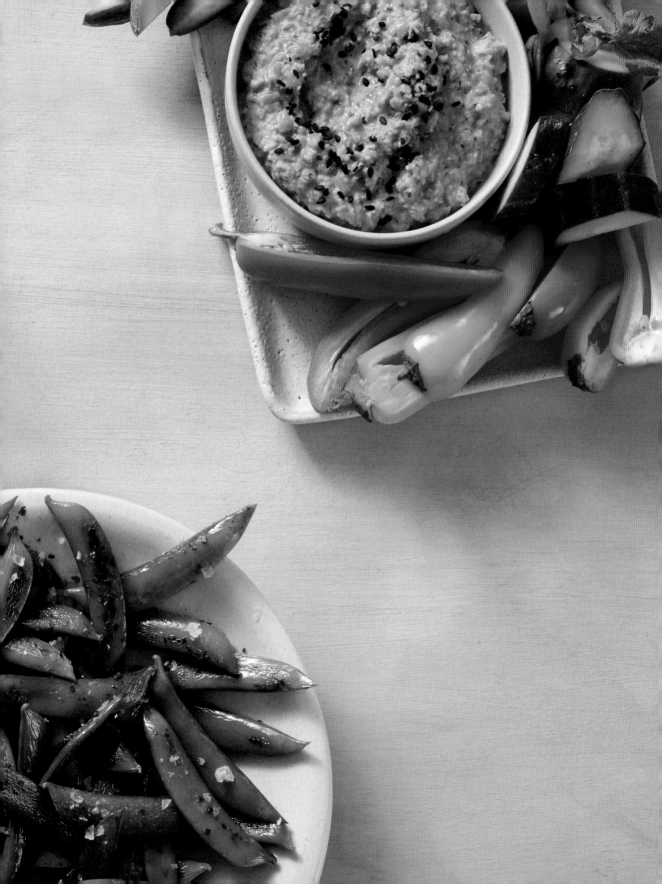

BLISTERED SUGAR SNAP PEAS 🌱

TOTAL TIME: 10 MINUTES ◆ SERVES 4

Sugar snap peas are good on their own, but a little char, zingy lime, and flaky salt push them to the next level—all while preserving their natural vitamin A content.

1 teaspoon olive oil

1 pound sugar snap peas, strings discarded

¼ teaspoon ground Aleppo pepper

1 teaspoon lime zest

1 tablespoon lime juice

½ teaspoon flaky sea salt

1. Heat a large cast-iron skillet on high. Add 1 teaspoon oil and then, in 2 batches, sugar sugar snap peas. Cook, tossing once, until bright green and charred and blistered in spots, 3 minutes. Transfer to a bowl; repeat.

2. Toss cooked sugar snap peas with Aleppo pepper and lime zest and juice. Sprinkle with sea salt.

PER SERVING 35 calories, 1.5 g fat (0 g saturated fat), 2 g protein, 295 mg sodium, 5 g carbohydrates, 2 g fiber, 2.5 g sugars (0 g added sugars), 0 mg cholesterol

SWEET PEA DIP 🌱

TOTAL 10 MINUTES ◆ SERVES 6

Frozen vegetables offer convenience and a high concentration of nutrients. This recipe uses frozen peas to make a springy dip for fresh in-season veggies.

10 ounces frozen peas, thawed

¾ cup mint leaves

¼ cup tahini

2 teaspoons lemon zest

3 tablespoons lemon juice

½ clove garlic, grated

½ teaspoon salt

Black pepper

½ teaspoon extra virgin olive oil

½ teaspoon black sesame seeds

Sliced vegetables, for serving

1. In a food processor, puree peas, mint, tahini, lemon zest and juice, garlic, salt, and pepper until smooth, adding 1 tablespoon water at a time if mixture is too thick.

2. Transfer dip to a serving bowl. Top dip with oil and sesame seeds. Serve with vegetables for dipping. Makes 1½ cups.

PER SERVING 110 calories, 6 g fat (1 g saturated fat), 5 g protein, 220 mg sodium, 10 g carbohydrates, 4 g fiber, 2.5 g sugars (0 g added sugars), 0 mg cholesterol

MANGO ROLLS

TOTAL TIME: 30 MINUTES ◆ SERVES 4

Mango, rich in vitamins A and C, yields benefits for both a healthy immune system and complexion.

¼ cup sweet chili sauce

1 tablespoon rice vinegar

2 teaspoons fish sauce

1 teaspoon lime zest

1 tablespoon lime juice

8 rice spring roll wrappers

2 large carrots, peeled and cut into matchsticks

1 English cucumber, cut into matchsticks

1 large red pepper, seeded and cut into matchsticks

1 mango, thinly sliced

4 ounces small romaine lettuce leaves

½ cup mint leaves

½ cup cilantro leaves

1. In a small bowl, whisk together sweet chili sauce, vinegar, fish sauce, and lime zest and juice; set aside.

2. Add hot water to a large, shallow dish and submerge 1 wrapper in water to soften, 10 to 15 seconds. Transfer wrapper to a slightly damp surface and gently smooth it out into a circle. Repeat with another wrapper, placing it on top of the first.

3. Add about an eighth of carrot, cucumber, pepper, mango, and romaine to bottom third of wrappers and top with a few herb leaves. Fold bottoms of wrappers over filling, then gently roll and tuck wrappers over filling to cover. Fold in sides to seal, then roll until completely sealed.

4. Repeat process until all fillings are used, keeping assembled rolls covered with a damp towel. Cut rolls in half and serve with chili dipping sauce.

PER SERVING 235 calories, 1 g fat (0 g saturated fat), 5 g protein, 605 mg sodium, 53 g carbohydrates, 6 g fiber, 25.5 g sugars (9.5 g added sugars), 0 mg cholesterol

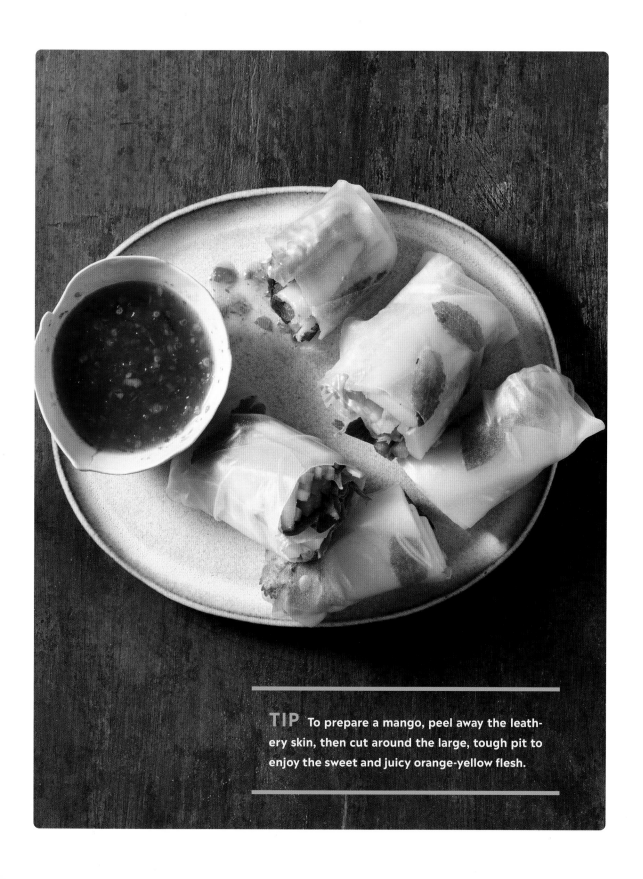

TIP To prepare a mango, peel away the leathery skin, then cut around the large, tough pit to enjoy the sweet and juicy orange-yellow flesh.

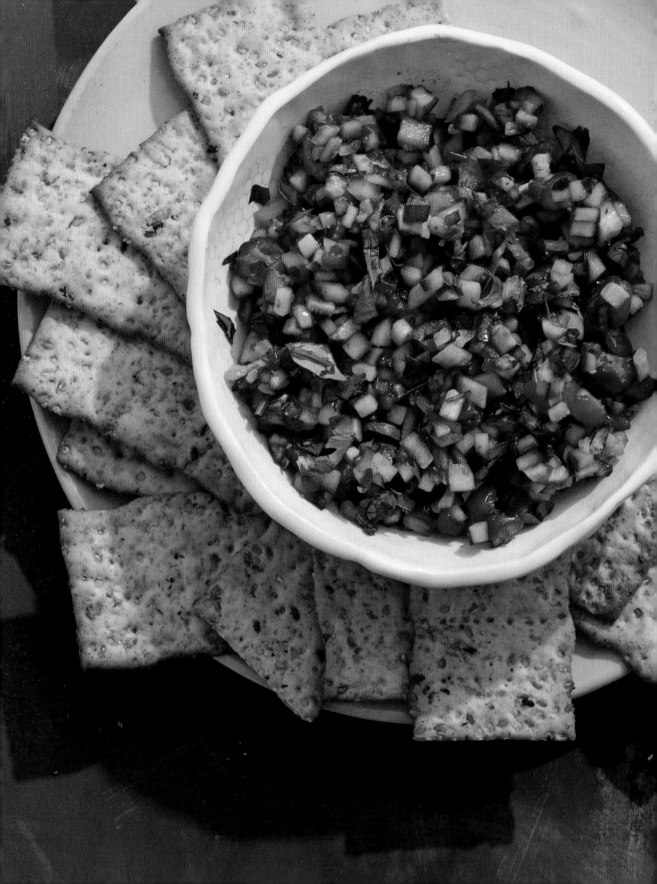

CRANBERRY SALSA

TOTAL TIME: 10 MINUTES ◆ SERVES 4

This unique take on salsa is sweet and spicy, featuring immune-boosting cranberries, refreshing cucumber, and spicy jalapeño.

1 cup fresh or frozen cranberries

1 Persian cucumber, finely chopped

½ small jalapeño, finely chopped

¼ sweet onion, finely chopped

¼ cup cilantro, finely chopped

1 teaspoon honey

½ teaspoon kosher salt

Crackers, for serving

1. In a food processor, pulse cranberries to finely chop. Transfer to a bowl.

2. Add cucumber, jalapeño, onion, and cilantro to the bowl with cranberries. Stir in honey and salt. Serve with crackers.

PER SERVING (salsa only): 30 calories, 0 g fat (0 g saturated fat), 0 g protein, 245 mg sodium, 7 g carbohydrates, 1 g fiber, 4 g sugars (1.5 g added sugars), 0 mg cholesterol

MAPLE-ROASTED BEETS

TOTAL TIME: 1 HOUR 5 MINUTES ◆ SERVES 6

You need only a touch of maple syrup to coax out the sweetness of these rich beets, which can help lower blood pressure and fight inflammation.

1 pound small beets, scrubbed and trimmed

2 tablespoons maple syrup

1 tablespoon olive oil

1 tablespoon orange juice

3 sprigs thyme

¼ teaspoon salt

¼ teaspoon black pepper

2 tablespoons lemon juice

Goat cheese or feta, crumbled, for topping

1. Heat oven to 450°F. In an 8-inch square baking pan, toss beets with maple syrup, oil, orange juice, thyme, ¼ cup water, salt, and pepper.

2. Wrap the pan tightly with foil, and roast the beets until tender, 40 to 45 minutes. Reserve beet cooking liquid.

3. Using a kitchen towel, lightly rub beets to remove skin. (It should come off easily—if not, beets are undercooked.) Cut into wedges; skewer, if desired.

4. In a bowl, whisk together lemon juice and 1½ tablespoons reserved beet liquid. Drizzle over beets and top with cheese.

PER SERVING 35 calories, 0.5 g fat (0 g saturated fat), 1 g protein, 60 mg sodium, 6 g carbohydrates, 1 g fiber, 4.5 g sugars (1 g added sugars), 0 mg cholesterol

TIP If a label says "pancake syrup," leave it on the shelf, as that means it's made mainly from corn syrup, colorings, flavorings, and preservatives. Real maple syrup has only one ingredient listed.

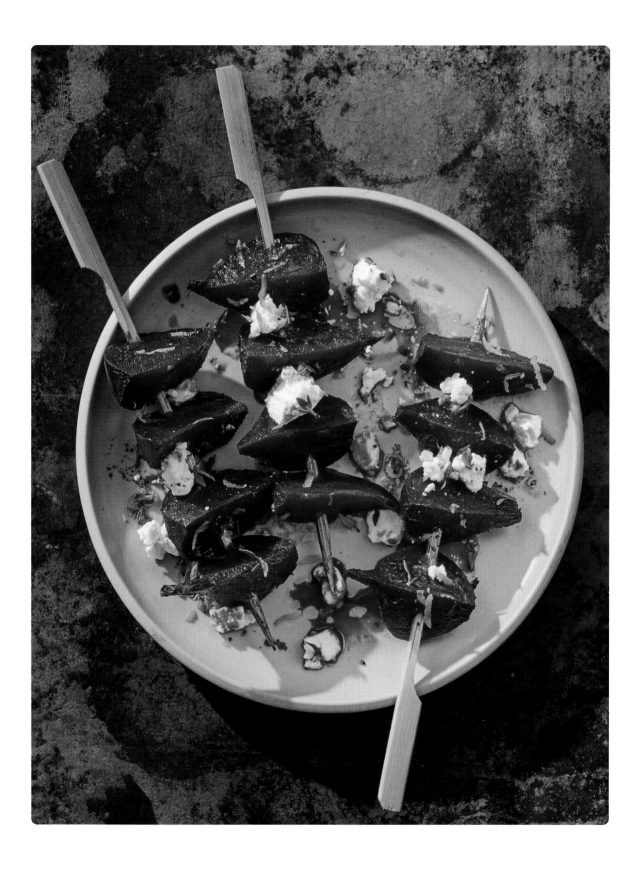

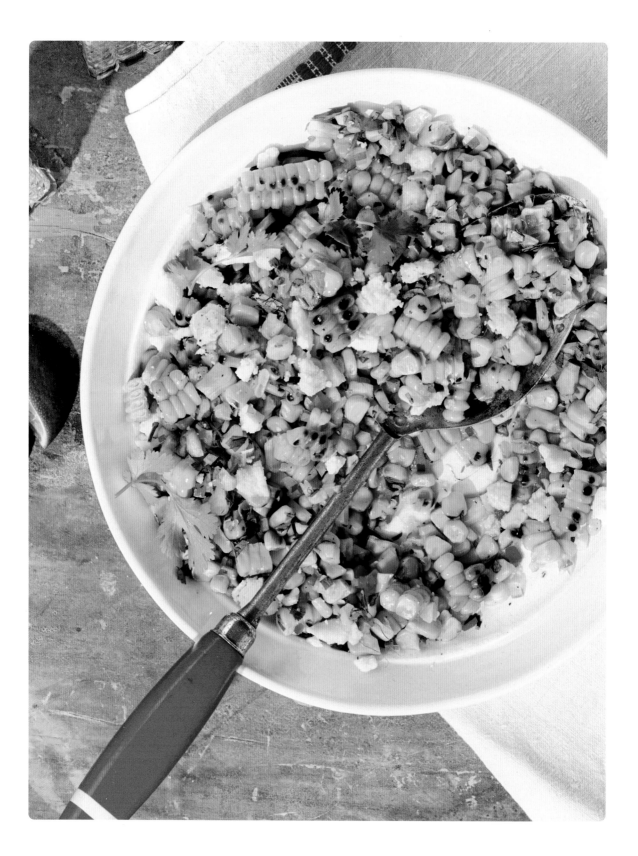

CHARRED CORN SALAD

TOTAL TIME: 35 MINUTES ◆ SERVES 8

Corn is one of the world's most popular cereal grains and a good source of vitamins such as B6, folate, and potassium. A little char on these cobs is an epic addition to this salad.

½ small red onion, finely chopped

1 red chile, seeded and chopped

¼ cup lime juice

1 tablespoon olive oil

Kosher salt

Black pepper

6 ears corn, shucked

¾ cup cilantro, chopped

3 ounces queso fresco, crumbled

1. Heat grill on medium. In a bowl, toss red onion, chile, lime juice, oil, and ½ teaspoon each salt and pepper.

2. Grill corn, turning occasionally, until charred, 10 to 12 minutes. Let cool, then cut corn from cobs.

3. Add to onion mixture and toss to combine. Fold in cilantro and queso fresco.

PER SERVING 130 calories, 6 g fat (2.5 g saturated fat), 5 g protein, 240 mg sodium, 16 g carbohydrates, 2 g fiber, 5.5 g sugars (0 g added sugars), 10 mg cholesterol

SMOKY GUACAMOLE 🌱

TOTAL TIME: 15 MINUTES   ◆   SERVES 5

This recipe brings a new, smoky flavor to the popular dip by charring the avocados first. Avocados are a great source of fiber, healthy fat, potassium, and vitamin C, which helps reduce skin inflammation, accelerate wound healing, and soothe dry skin.

2 ripe avocados, halved and pitted

2 teaspoons vegetable oil

3 tablespoons lime juice

½ teaspoon ground chipotle chile

½ teaspoon kosher salt

¼ cup finely chopped red onion

¼ cup cilantro, finely chopped

Tortilla chips, for serving

1. Heat grill on medium-high. Brush cut sides of avocados with oil. Grill just until slightly charred, 2 to 4 minutes.

2. Transfer avocados to cutting board and cool slightly. Scoop avocado into a bowl and mash with lime juice, ground chile, and salt.

3. Fold in red onion and cilantro. Serve with tortilla chips.

PER SERVING 150 calories, 13.5 g fat (2 g saturated fat), 2 g protein, 210 mg sodium, 9 g carbohydrates, 6 g fiber, 1 g sugars (0 g added sugars), 0 mg cholesterol

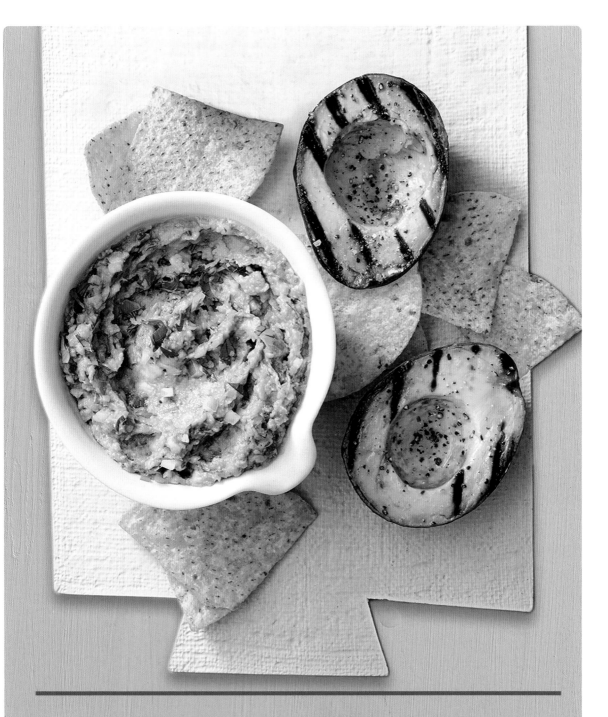

TIP Without enough potassium in your diet, you can drink all the water you want but you won't be well hydrated. Forget bananas—avocados are a top source of this mineral too.

JALAPEÑO-POBLANO SALSA VERDE 🌱

This charred salsa verde is a low-calorie treat. While it's tasty enough to stand on its own, you can add zing to your weeknight dinners (literally) by using a little of this salsa to top everything from salads to sandwiches.

1 jalapeño, seeded and chopped

½ small red onion, finely chopped

2 tablespoons lime juice

Kosher salt

3 large poblano chiles (about 11 ounces)

1 green pepper

1 tablespoon olive oil

½ cup cilantro leaves, finely chopped

Romaine lettuce hearts, for serving

1. Place oven rack in upper third of oven; heat broiler. In a small bowl, toss jalapeño, onion, lime juice, and a pinch of salt; let sit.

2. Halve and seed remaining peppers. Arrange on a rimmed baking sheet, cut side down. Drizzle with oil. Broil until charred, 10 minutes. Cool, scrape off skin, and coarsely chop. Stir into onion mixture along with cilantro. Serve with lettuce.

PER SERVING 30 calories, 1.5 g fat (0 g saturated fat), 1 g protein, 20 mg sodium, 6 g carbohydrates, 1 g fiber, 1 g sugars (0 g added sugars), 0 mg cholesterol

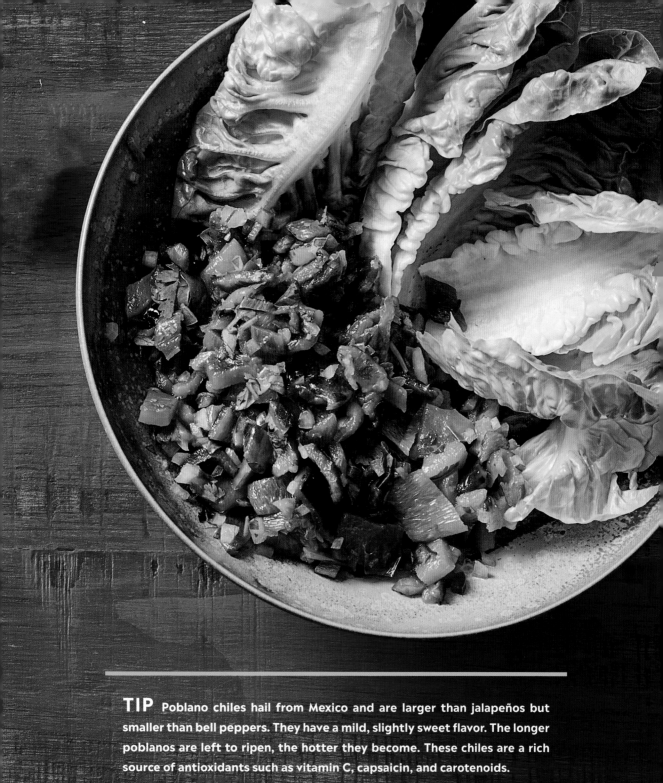

TIP Poblano chiles hail from Mexico and are larger than jalapeños but smaller than bell peppers. They have a mild, slightly sweet flavor. The longer poblanos are left to ripen, the hotter they become. These chiles are a rich source of antioxidants such as vitamin C, capsaicin, and carotenoids.

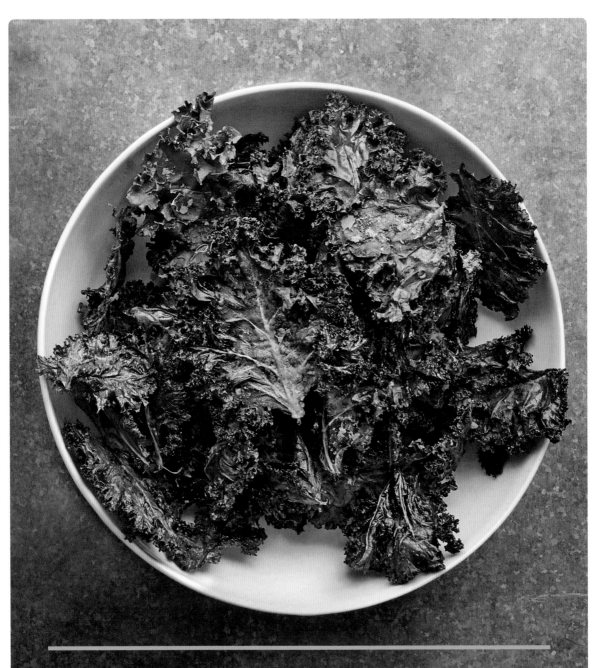

TIP There are two nutritional yeast product offerings to choose from when shopping. Unfortified means it's plain yeast without any additives, while fortified includes added vitamins and minerals. Both toppings are healthy choices.

"CHEESY" KALE CHIPS 🌱

TOTAL TIME: 35 MINUTES ◆ SERVES 2

Nutritional yeast, rich in B vitamins and protein, is a tasty and "cheesy" addition to these crunchy cruciferous chips, a dairy-free snack.

1 small bunch kale

1 tablespoon olive oil

2 tablespoons nutritional yeast flakes

¼ teaspoon kosher salt

1. Heat oven to 325°F. Rinse kale, pat very dry with paper towels, and remove thick stems and discard. Tear leaves into similarly sized pieces.

2. Place on a baking sheet, drizzle with oil, and toss to coat. Sprinkle with nutritional yeast and salt; toss to coat.

3. Bake, tossing twice, until kale chips are crisp, 25 to 30 minutes. Let cool 5 minutes before serving.

PER SERVING 120 calories, 8 g fat (1 g saturated fat), 7 g protein, 275 mg sodium, 9 g carbohydrates, 3 g fiber, 0 g sugars (0 g added sugars), 0 mg cholesterol

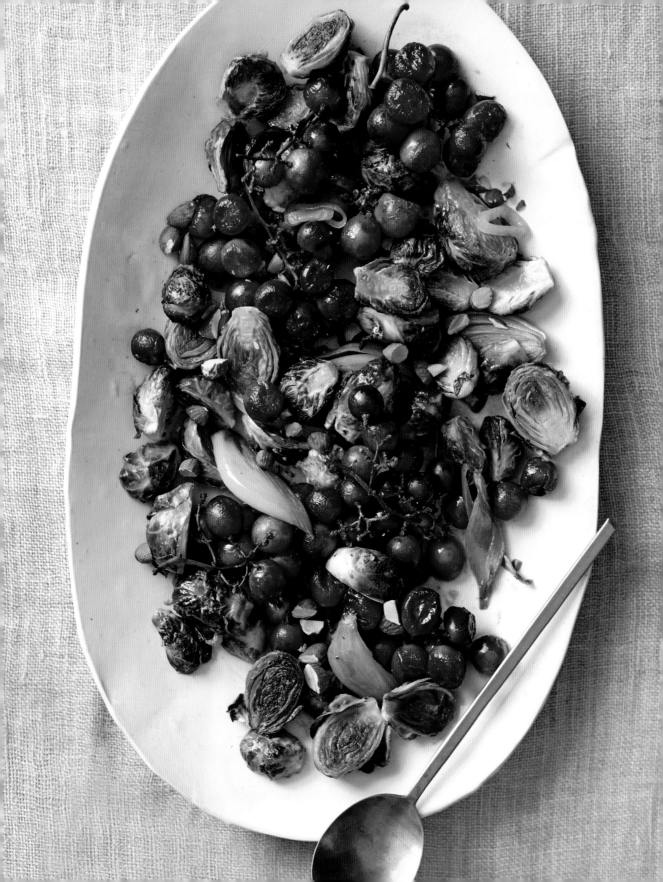

ROASTED BRUSSELS SPROUTS WITH GRAPES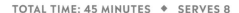

TOTAL TIME: 45 MINUTES ◆ SERVES 8

Prepare this recipe in the winter when Brussels sprouts and grapes are in season. This side dish is the verdant antidote to a chilly evening.

1½ pounds Brussels sprouts, trimmed and halved

3 tablespoons olive oil, divided

½ teaspoon kosher salt

¼ teaspoon black pepper

3 large shallots, cut in ¼-inch slices

2 cups seedless red grapes

1 tablespoon red wine vinegar

⅛ cup roasted unsalted almonds, coarsely chopped, for topping

1. Heat oven to 425°F. On a rimmed baking sheet, toss Brussels sprouts with 2 tablespoons oil, salt, and pepper.

2. On a separate rimmed baking sheet, toss shallots and grapes with remaining 1 tablespoon oil. Transfer both sheets to oven and roast, stirring grapes after 15 minutes and turning Brussels sprouts after 20 minutes, until sprouts are golden brown and tender, 25 to 35 minutes total.

3. Combine vinegar with 1 tablespoon water and toss with grapes, stirring and scraping up any browned bits. Toss grape mixture and sprouts together and top with almonds.

PER SERVING 150 calories, 8 g fat (1 g saturated fat), 4 g protein, 140 mg sodium, 17 g carbohydrates, 4 g fiber, 9 g sugars (0 g added sugars), 0 mg cholesterol

ROASTED VEGGIES WITH OLIVE DRESSING

TOTAL TIME: 55 MINUTES ◆ **SERVES 10**

Parsnips are the star of this hearty side. This root vegetable provides plenty of fiber and potassium, both of which will keep you energized long after your meal ends.

2 pounds parsnips, peeled, thin ends trimmed away, halved or quartered lengthwise

5 tablespoons extra virgin olive oil, divided

2 teaspoons kosher salt, divided

2 pounds sweet potatoes, peeled, ends trimmed, cut lengthwise into wedges

3 tablespoons lemon juice

½ small shallot, finely chopped

1 small clove garlic, finely chopped

½ cup pitted black, green, or kalamata olives (or a combination), coarsely chopped

½ cup loosely packed mint leaves, coarsely chopped, for topping

½ cup cilantro leaves, coarsely chopped, for topping

1. Heat oven to 375°F. On a rimmed baking sheet, toss parsnips with 1 tablespoon oil and 1 teaspoon salt; arrange in single layer and roast 10 minutes.

2. Meanwhile, on a second baking sheet, toss sweet potatoes with 1 tablespoon oil and 1 teaspoon salt; arrange in single layer.

3. Toss parsnips; return to oven along with potatoes and roast, stirring vegetables after 25 minutes, until golden brown and tender, 40 to 50 minutes total.

4. Meanwhile, make vinaigrette: In a small bowl, combine lemon juice, shallot, garlic, and remaining 3 tablespoons oil. Stir in olives. When ready to serve, transfer vegetables to a platter and spoon dressing on top. Sprinkle with mint and cilantro. Serve warm or at room temperature.

PER SERVING 195 calories, 9 g fat (1 g saturated fat), 2 g protein, 270 mg sodium, 28 g carbohydrates, 6 g fiber, 8 g sugars (0 g added sugars), 0 mg cholesterol

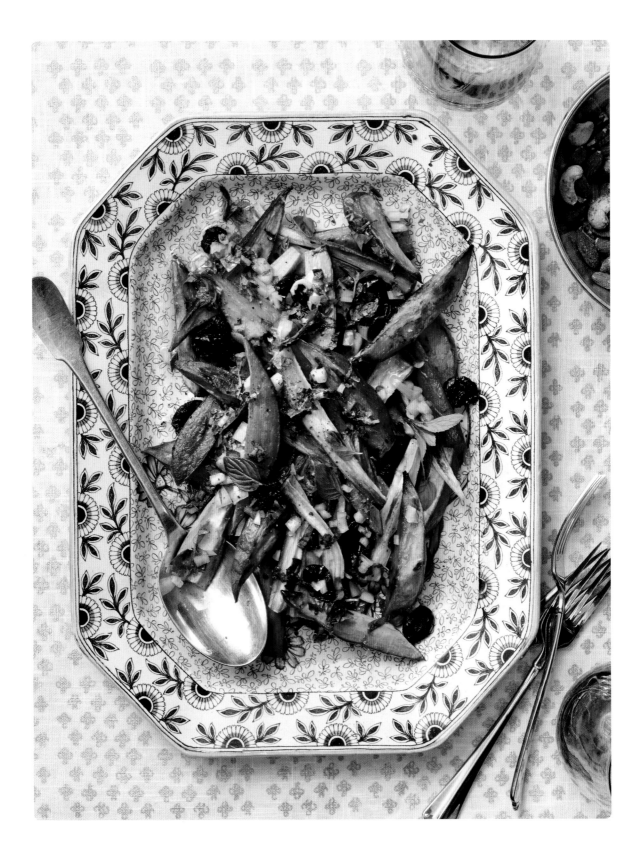

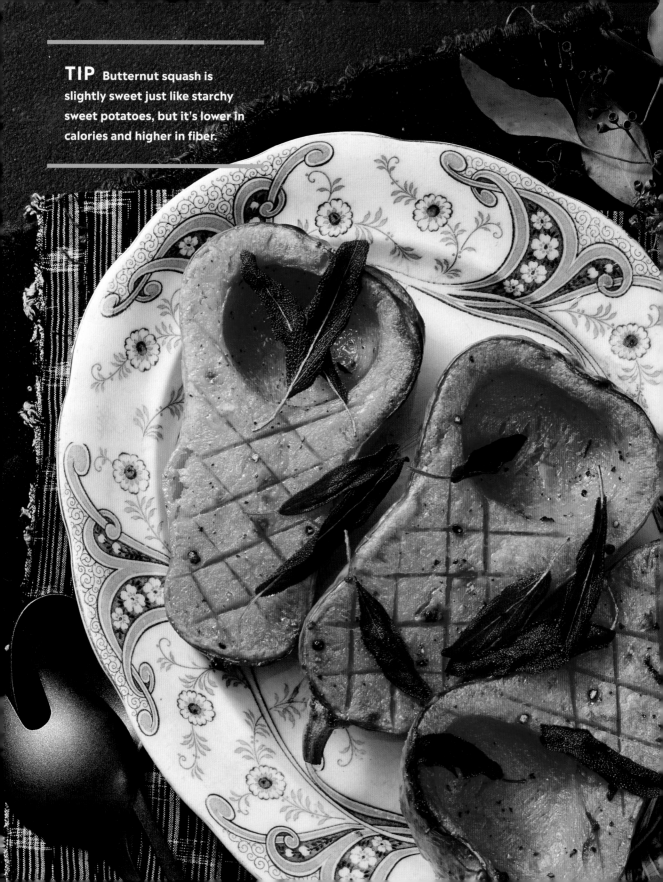

TIP Butternut squash is slightly sweet just like starchy sweet potatoes, but it's lower in calories and higher in fiber.

ROASTED BUTTERNUT SQUASH WITH FRIZZLED SAGE ❧

Just one serving of this side provides half of your daily vitamin C and more than 100 percent of your daily vitamin A, mainly in the form of beta-carotene, which may help protect your cells.

⅓ cup olive oil, plus more for the baking sheet

⅓ cup sage leaves

2 small butternut squash (about 2 pounds each)

¾ teaspoon kosher salt

¼ teaspoon black pepper

1. Heat oven to 400°F. Line a rimmed baking sheet with foil; oil the foil.

2. Heat ⅓ cup oil in a small saucepan on medium. Add sage leaves and cook, stirring, until bubbling subsides and leaves are crisp, about 1 minute. Transfer leaves to a paper-towel-lined plate; reserve oil.

3. Cut butternut squash in half lengthwise; scoop out and discard seeds. Using a sharp paring knife, score the flesh of the neck of the squash in a crisscross pattern. Working on the prepared baking sheet, coat squash with 2 tablespoons reserved oil and season with salt and pepper.

4. Place squash cut side down and roast in lower half of oven until flesh begins to turn golden brown, 30 to 35 minutes. Turn squash and roast until skin is golden brown and crisp, 45 to 55 minutes more. Serve topped with crispy sage leaves.

PER SERVING 125 calories, 4.5 g fat (0.5 g saturated fat), 2 g protein, 190 mg sodium, 23 g carbohydrates, 4 g fiber, 4 g sugars (0 g added sugars), 0 mg cholesterol

CORN ON THE COB WITH CHILI-LIME SAUCE

TOTAL TIME: 20 MINUTES ◆ SERVES 8

The antioxidants in corn can help strengthen your vision and may also help prevent hardening of the arteries. The chili-lime sauce is heart-healthy, and adding spice is a great trick for eating more slowly, preventing overeating.

½ cup extra virgin olive oil

1 small jalapeño, thinly sliced

¼ cup sour cream

2 tablespoons fat-free milk

8 ears corn, shucked

1½ teaspoons chili powder

½ teaspoon kosher salt

¼ cup chopped chives

8 lime wedges, for serving

1. In a small saucepan, bring oil and jalapeño to a simmer on medium heat. Remove from heat and let steep 10 minutes. In a bowl, whisk together sour cream and milk.

2. Bring a large pot of salted water to a boil. Add corn and cook until bright yellow and tender, 3 minutes. Remove from water. Drizzle with half the jalapeño-oil mixture and sprinkle with chili powder and salt. Toss corn to coat, adding more of the mixture if necessary. Top with sour cream sauce and chives, and serve with lime wedges.

PER SERVING 230 calories, 16.5 g fat (3 g saturated fat), 4 g protein, 140 mg sodium, 20 g carbohydrates, 2 g fiber, 7 g sugars (0 g added sugars), 3 mg cholesterol

TIP To choose the freshest corn, look for bright-green husks, kernels that are firm and close together, and tassels that are brown and sticky.

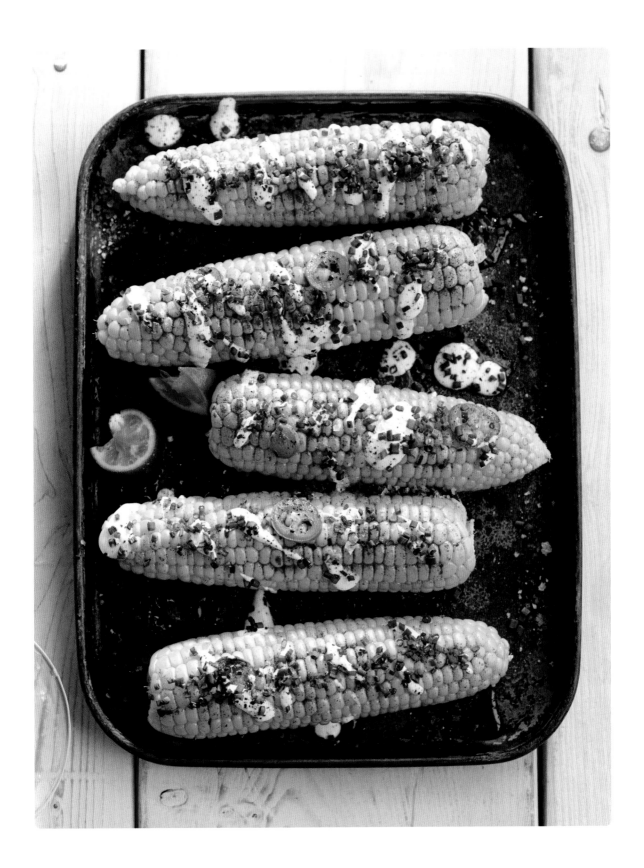

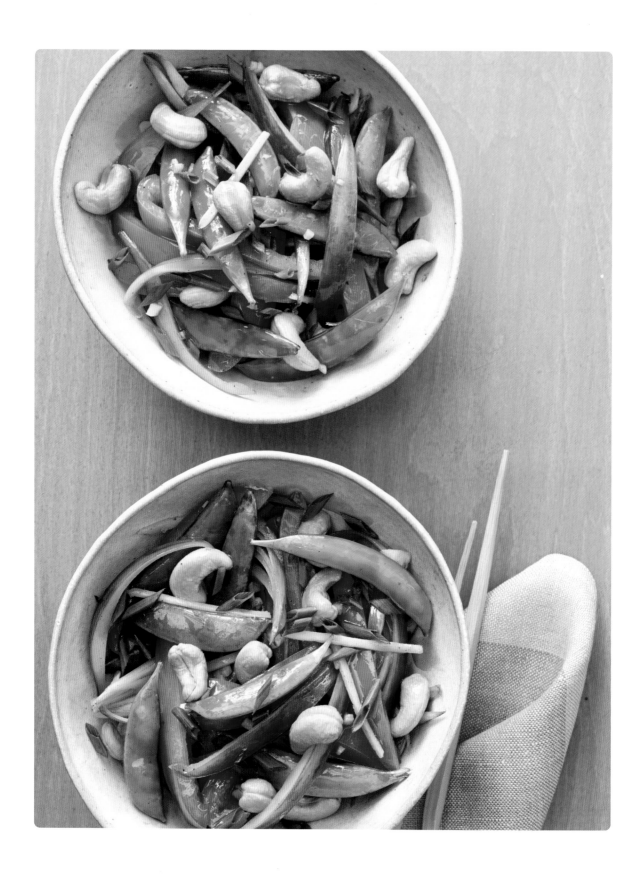

CASHEW & PEPPER STIR-FRY

TOTAL TIME: 20 MINUTES ◆ SERVES 4

Protein-packed cashews add crunch while anti-inflammatory ginger, sweet honey, and fragrant onion add flavor to this delicious side dish. Want to make it a main meal? Toss in your favorite alternative protein source. It's that simple.

3 tablespoons reduced-sodium soy sauce

1 tablespoon seasoned rice vinegar

2 teaspoons cornstarch

2 teaspoons honey

2 teaspoons vegetable oil

2 cloves garlic, minced

1 (½-inch) piece ginger, peeled and cut into matchsticks

1 cup sugar snap peas, trimmed

1 large red pepper, sliced

1 medium red onion, sliced into ½-inch wedges

6 tablespoons roasted cashews, for topping

Sliced chives, for topping

1. Combine soy sauce, vinegar, cornstarch, and honey.

2. Heat oil in a skillet on high. Add garlic and ginger; cook until lightly browned, 1 minute. Add peas, pepper, and onion. Cook, stirring occasionally, until crisp-tender, 3 minutes.

3. Add sauce mixture and cook until slightly thickened, 30 seconds. Serve topped with cashews and chives.

PER SERVING 155 calories, 8.5 g fat (1.5 g saturated fat), 4 g protein, 405 mg sodium, 17 g carbohydrates, 3 g fiber, 8 g sugars (1 g added sugars), 0 mg cholesterol

HEARTY BRUSSELS SPROUT SLAW 🌱

TOTAL TIME: 25 MINUTES ◆ SERVES 16

Coleslaw can easily become mundane, so why not switch up the crunchy green base vegetable? Brussels sprouts contain powerful antioxidants, which are helpful in repairing and preventing free-radical damage to your cells.

1½ cups extra virgin olive oil

1 cup apple cider vinegar

4 teaspoons Dijon mustard

2 small shallots, minced

1 teaspoon kosher salt

1 teaspoon black pepper

2 pounds Brussels sprouts, trimmed and shredded

2 (10-ounce) bags frozen shelled edamame, thawed

2 cups parsley leaves

2 cups pomegranate arils

1 cup chopped walnuts, toasted

1. To a 1-quart jar with lid, add oil, vinegar, mustard, shallots, salt, and pepper; shake until combined.

2. Toss sprouts, edamame, parsley, and pomegranate with 1 cup or more of dressing. Serve with walnuts or cover and store for up to 5 days in refrigerator.

PER SERVING 200 calories, 13 g fat (1.5 g saturated fat), 7 g protein, 75 mg sodium, 15 g carbohydrates, 5 g fiber, 5 g sugars (0 g added sugars), 0 mg cholesterol

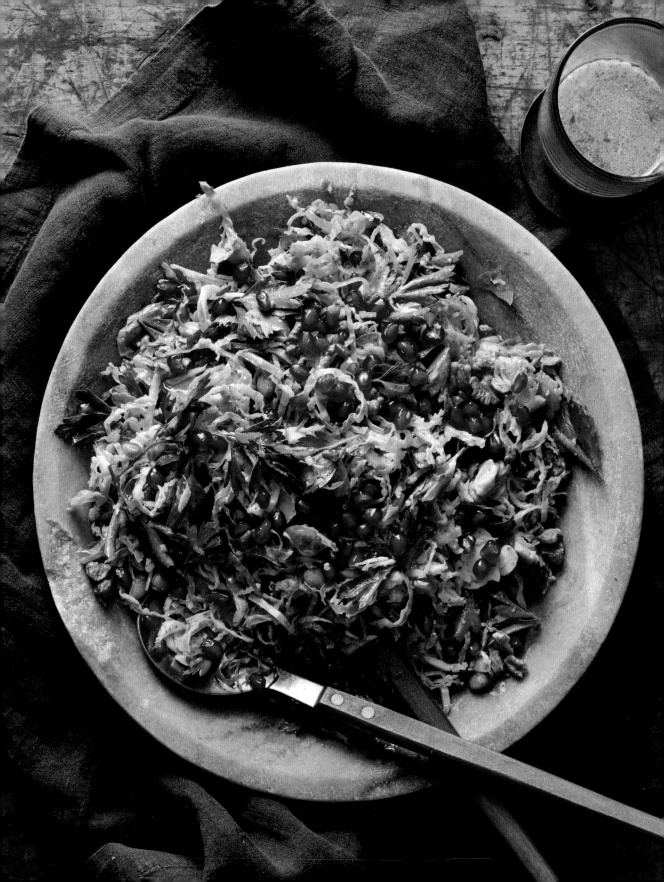

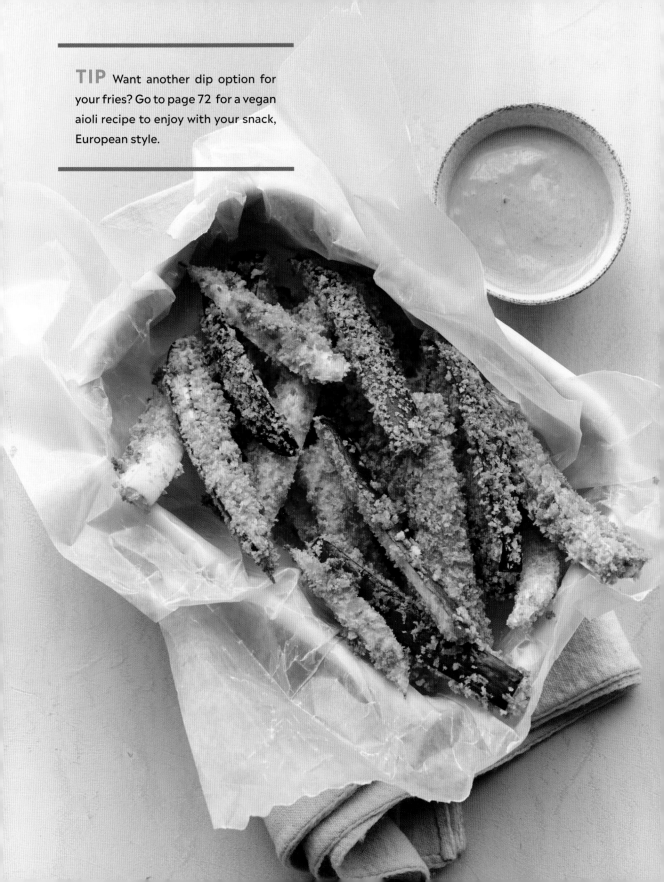

TIP Want another dip option for your fries? Go to page 72 for a vegan aioli recipe to enjoy with your snack, European style.

EGGPLANT & ZUCCHINI FRIES WITH ROASTED TOMATO DIP

TOTAL TIME: 1 HOUR ◆ SERVES 8

We all crave fries every once in a while. This recipe will let you indulge without compromising on nutrition. Make sure to cut the squash, zucchini, and eggplant into similarly sized pieces so they cook evenly in the oven.

1 cup cherry tomatoes

1 teaspoon olive oil

1 cup plain fat-free Greek yogurt

2 teaspoons apple cider vinegar

½ teaspoon Dijon mustard

½ teaspoon kosher salt, divided

½ teaspoon black pepper, divided

5 large egg whites, beaten

2½ cups panko breadcrumbs, toasted

1 medium yellow squash

1 medium zucchini

1 small eggplant

1. Heat oven to 375°F. On a baking sheet, toss tomatoes and oil; roast 15 minutes.

2. In a food processor, puree roasted tomatoes with yogurt, vinegar, mustard, and ¼ teaspoon each salt and pepper. Transfer to a bowl and chill.

3. Place egg whites in a dish. In a separate dish, mix breadcrumbs with remaining ¼ teaspoon each salt and pepper.

4. Cut vegetables into ½-inch-thick fries. Dip in egg whites, roll in breadcrumbs, and place on a separate baking sheet.

5. Bake until golden, 15 to 18 minutes. Serve with dip.

PER SERVING 240 calories, 2.5 g fat (0 g saturated fat), 15 g protein, 355 mg sodium, 41 g carbohydrates, 4 g fiber, 10 g sugars (0 g added sugars), 1 mg cholesterol

APPLE ENERGY BALLS

TOTAL TIME: 10 MINUTES ◆ SERVES 12

Perfect as a quick midmorning snack or an afternoon pick-me-up, these fiber- and antioxidant-filled apple bites are easy to transport and will keep the doctor, well, you know where.

1 cup dried apples, chopped

6 pitted Medjool dates

1 tablespoon honey

½ teaspoon cinnamon

¼ teaspoon ground nutmeg

¼ teaspoon salt

½ cup toasted walnuts

1. In a food processor, puree dried apples, dates, honey, cinnamon, nutmeg, and salt until almost smooth.

2. Add walnuts and pulse to incorporate. Firmly roll into 1-inch balls. Refrigerate at least 2 hours and up to 5 days.

PER SERVING 75 calories, 2.5 g fat (0.5 g saturated fat), 1 g protein, 15 mg sodium, 14 g carbohydrates, 2 g fiber, 11.5 g sugars (1.5 g added sugars), 0 mg cholesterol

TIP Try different kinds of dried apples in this recipe. Honeycrisp or Gala apples will add sweetness, while green apples offer more tart and complex flavors.

OLIVE TAPENADE

TOTAL TIME: 10 MINUTES ◆ SERVES 4

Beat bloat with this umami-rich, heart-healthy spread: All olives are low in FODMAPs, a type of carbohydrate that can be tough on digestion. Here, the Provençal-style appetizer is served with crackers, but it would also make a flavorful topping for a plant-based protein.

1 cup baby spinach

½ cup pitted kalamata olives

¼ cup canned sliced water chestnuts, drained

3 oil-packed anchovies, drained

2 tablespoons hulled sunflower seeds

2 tablespoons chopped parsley

1 tablespoon olive oil

1 tablespoon capers, drained

1 teaspoon Dijon mustard

1 teaspoon lemon juice

Plain rice crackers, for serving

1. In a food processor, pulse spinach, olives, water chestnuts, anchovies, sunflower seeds, parsley, olive oil, capers, mustard, and lemon juice to coarsely chop.

2. Serve with small plain rice crackers.

PER SERVING 280 calories, 19 g fat (2.5 g saturated fat), 5 g protein, 970 mg sodium, 23 g carbohydrates, 2 g fiber, 1 g sugars (0 g added sugars), 0 mg cholesterol

TIP Experiment with which olives you like best for this dish. You can use buttery or spicy kalamata olives or even briny green olives in the mix. Just make sure to buy pitted olives before tossing them into a food processor.

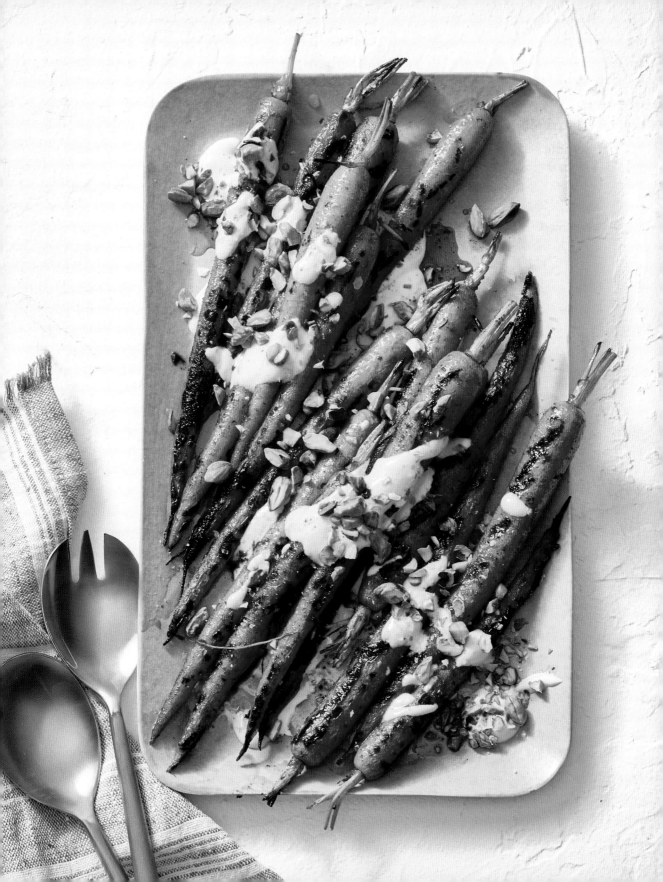

GRILLED CARROTS

TOTAL TIME: 25 MINUTES ◆ SERVES 6

The combo of creamy Greek yogurt and tahini—a savory condiment made with sesame seeds—adds some tang to smoky, spicy carrots.

2 bunches thin carrots with tops, scrubbed and trimmed

1 tablespoon olive oil

2 teaspoons honey

1 teaspoon harissa

¼ cup plain 2-percent Greek yogurt

2 tablespoons tahini

2 tablespoons lemon juice

¼ teaspoon kosher salt

¼ teaspoon black pepper

2 tablespoons pistachios, toasted and finely chopped

1. Heat grill on low. Halve any large carrots lengthwise if needed, to ensure that all carrots are of similar thickness. In a large bowl, whisk together oil, honey, and harissa. Add carrots and toss to coat.

2. Place carrots on grill (perpendicular to grates) and grill, covered, rolling or turning halfway through, until charred and tender, 10 to 12 minutes. Transfer to a platter.

3. Meanwhile, in a bowl, whisk together yogurt, tahini, lemon juice, salt, and pepper. Gradually drizzle in 2 tablespoons warm water, adding more if mixture seems too thick. Drizzle over carrots, and sprinkle with pistachios.

PER SERVING 110 calories, 6.5 g fat (1 g saturated fat), 3 g protein, 135 mg sodium, 11 g carbohydrates, 3 g fiber, 7 g sugars (2 g added sugars), 1 mg cholesterol

INDEX